I am so thankful that I met Donna and followed her dietary advice. As a result, I was able to attain my childhood dream of becoming a model, and I did it in my mid-forties.

279-3663

Arlene, East Greenbush, NY

As a postal carrier, the excess weight I gained took its toll on my body. My knees hurt every day until I went to Donna and lost thirty-two pounds. She taught me how to make dietary substitutions that actually made me feel as if I wasn't dieting. I can say without any shadow of a doubt that Donna's diet always delivers results!

Paul, Albany, NY

I went on the Net Calorie Diet prior to entering a beauty pageant. I lost weight and then won Miss Albany.

Anna, East Greenbush, NY

I've always wanted to compete in a marathon, but I weighed too much to be able to endure a twenty-six-mile race. My friends recommended that I join Donna's diet program. I followed her diet and fitness instructions, which helped me to lose weight and build endurance. Then I entered my first marathon, and the moment I crossed the finish line I felt happier than I ever have in my entire life.

Maryann, Pittstown, NY

I joined the Net Calorie Diet to lose twenty pounds and help alleviate my arthritis. I stayed on the diet after my twenty-pound loss because I've never felt better. I wouldn't call myself an athlete, but due to Donna's encouragement, I entered the empire state games. She put me on an exercise program. Donna even took the time to personally train with me and cheer me on at the race. I won a gold medal at the empire state games, and I'm over fifty years old. My grandchildren are very proud of me. Thank you, Donna!

Delores, Troy, NY

When I started the program, I was on high blood pressure medication and high cholesterol drugs. I had joined a gym to try to lose weight, but my efforts were in vain. Then I met Donna and started her diet. I was losing weight, and I felt motivated. I even lost twelve pounds in one week. After I lost thirty pounds, I was able to stop taking all my prescription drugs. My daughter was so impressed that she joined the program. This program made me feel twenty years younger. I know how to keep the weight off, and I'm indebted to Donna for teaching me the skills to do so.

Jean, East Greenbush, NY

The thing I loved most about Donna's diet is that I could eat what I wanted and still lose weight. Donna actually cooked my family and me a pasta casserole during my diet meeting. The meal was so huge that I felt like I was cheating. The recipe became a family favorite ever since we first tasted it. I lost over thirty pounds and was able to stop taking my diabetes medication. I'm healthy and enjoying my retirement thanks to Donna.

John, Rennsselear, NY

I was diagnosed as a diabetic and had several intestinal disorders when I turned to Donna for help. It was soon thereafter that my blood sugar levels returned to normal and all my bowel problems ceased. I am a contractor, so it's vital that I maintain my stamina. After following this diet program, my workers were amazed that I am in better shape than men who are one-third my age. I'm over sixty-five now, and I compete in track and field events. I exercise every day and work over fifty hours a week. My energy level is unbelievable. It's better than when I was twenty years old! I am grateful that Donna is now going to be able to help millions of people feel as fit and trim as I do.

Robert, Mattydale, NY

I came to Donna after my friends lost weight on the program. I listened to her instructions and lost thirteen pounds my first week. It was amazing!

Bob, Grafton, NY

I've owned a workout center for many years and asked Donna to give a speech on weight loss. She was happy to oblige, and after her free seminar, my members were asking to join the diet. I was honored to give Donna an office at the club so that she could offer the program to my customers. The part that amazed me the most was that this was the only diet that I never received a single complaint about. In fact, it was commonplace for my members to compliment her diet and thank me for having Donna there to help with them.

Nick, Club East, East Greenbush, NY

I've been on numerous diets throughout my life, and I've never met anyone more dedicated to helping each and every client lose weight than Donna. When I first met Donna, I said to her, "I feel like I found a goldmine." It's like having your very own Diet Angel that protects you from sinful temptations.

Florence, Pleasantdale, NY

DEDICATION

This book is devoted to everyone who has ever stepped on a scale and not liked the number he or she has seen. This program is for the disgruntled dieters who have been lied to, deceived, and cheated. This book is for every person who was robbed of his or her hard-earned dollars by the false promises of fad diets, unscrupulous diet ads, and pseudo potions and pills. It's for the individual who goes through life trying diet after diet, and the lack of results leaves him or her feeling hopeless. You deserve your life back, which is just what this book can help you accomplish. I hope and pray that this book inspires you to achieve your weight loss goal and enriches every aspect of your life. Once your eyes have been opened, you will see that the road is paved with success. It is through knowledge, wisdom, and devotion that we acquire the power to attain the desires of our heart. May you look forward to each and every day without the burden of obesity in your way.

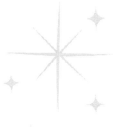

ACKNOWLEDGMENTS

My first thanks is to God for providing me with the wisdom, knowledge, and passion to help others. It's an honor to serve the Lord in such a worldwide capacity.

I am indebted to my loving and patient husband. He put my daily handwritten words into orderly chapters. Bill sat and eagerly listened when I read back my text to make sure it was witty and informative. He spent many hours at the computer correcting typographical errors and putting over one hundred tables and charts into order. Bill found typing errors that evaded editors and proofreaders, which proves that a loving eye can see beyond the written word. I will say that words alone cannot express my gratitude for all the hard work he put into this book. I'm confident I'll find other ways of showing my appreciation!

I would like to thank my brother-in-law Bob for his expert proofreading and editing. I must say that writing a book is rather intoxicating. Although the editing phase is most assuredly sobering, it's enlightening to have an in-law who's not afraid to be honest. As I constantly remind Bob, the errors were probably made by the typist and not by the author.

I am in appreciation of my brother-in-law Randy Masters. He is my big-shot New York City 5th Avenue lawyer. The man who looked over my contracts and provided trustworthy counsel. I of course received a generous pro bono family discount.

I am deeply grateful to Tate publishing for giving me the opportunity to tell the world the truth about dieting. When Trinity Tate sent me my contract, she put two handwritten words at the bottom of the acceptance letter. They are the words every author waits to hear: great book! It brought tears to my eyes, because I knew my twenty-two years of painstaking research were coming to fruition. I was treated like family from the moment I signed on with Tate Publishing.

My heartfelt thanks go out to Meghan Barnes, my editor. Her eye for detail is appreciated. I was impressed with the fact that she included her individual thoughts and comments throughout the manuscript. She sets high standards, and I wouldn't want it any other way. I thank her for the compliments and encouraging emails. The one particular e-mail that keeps coming to mind is when Meghan reminded me that we want this book to be perfect. I thank you for your time and devotion to this endeavor.

I would like to thank Lindsay Behrens, my graphic designer, for her patience. She worked diligently at achieving a stunning front cover. It's a fact that one customer stated she would buy the book because of its beautiful cover. The goal was to create a cartoon that represented me, the diet lady. The finished product is eye catching and is sure to attract everyone's attention.

I thank my immediate family, which includes Mom C., Mom W., Ron, Dad M., Dad B., and my new family, my brother Joe and his son, Joe, my sister Sheila and her beloved family. I would like to also thank my extended family and friends (which includes the A.B.C.) for their prayers and inspiration throughout this entire process. Your kind words provided incentive for me to put my words into a bestseller. I pray that God eternally blesses everyone who helped me!

TABLE OF CONTENTS

FOREWORD

It's a battlefield out there, where you have to fight for your right to be thin and corporate giants wait to prey upon innocent dieters. It's refreshing to know that there's a woman like Donna who brings integrity to the industry. I remember when Donna started writing this book she would share her ideas with us as the book progressed. Her enthusiasm was contagious, because our whole circle of friends became diet conscious. It was commonplace when we were out at art receptions to find Donna hovering over the buffet, giving out dietary advice. She is dedicated to solving worldwide obesity, because she knows the profound effects it has on people's lives. Her personal story is amazing! She proves that no matter what the circumstances are that no one is ever doomed to be over-weight. Her lifelong endeavor to conquer obesity provides positive encourage-ment to overcome the personal obstacles that stand in the way of achieving our weight loss goals. Donna's program in unique because she combines science and psychology and puts it all into lay terms. Her peerless metaphors and parables shed light onto the darkness of dieting. I am a firm believer in education, and Donna is the consummate diet teacher. There is valuable information to be learned in every chapter. Donna even included a special section on childhood obesity, which should be read by every parent. Donna's book covers every aspect of weight loss. She has the uncanny ability to make you smile, laugh, and diet simultaneously. This book fills you up with so much dietary knowledge that you will never hunger again. It's comforting to know that the world will finally know the truth about dieting. This is a must-read book for everyone who wants to take control of his or her weight and live a long, healthy life.

Dr. Joan W. Burns RN, MS, MS Ed, Ph.D
Ph.D. (Education)
Master of Science (Health Education)
Master of Science in Education (Educational Psychology)

ABOUT THE AUTHOR

Donna Masters was professionally educated at Syracuse University where she received two degrees, one in chemical engineering and the other in mathematics. Donna is the originator and owner of the Diet Research Clinic where she has been triumphantly counseling diet clients on a one-on-one basis for twenty-two years. Donna also owned and operated a natural food store called Brunswick Naturals for twelve years. In an effort to prove the benefits of this diet, Donna has competed in numerous sports events. She started her athletic endeavor by entering a bodybuilding contest and won first place. Donna moved onto power lifting where she won first place in every event she entered. It only took her a couple of months to break state and national records in her weight class. After Donna established her strength, she decided to challenge her speed. This was accomplished by becoming a race walker. On July 24, 2008, Donna won her tenth straight gold medal in the empire state games—and her time was faster than it was ten years ago—by walking over 6 miles an hour for 3.1 miles. She is now considered one of the fastest and strongest women in the country for her age and weight. It's important to note that Donna achieved these goals while she was running a natural food store, counseling her diet clients, inventing the net calorie, and writing a diet book. She unites her knowledge of science and the wisdom of her experience into a unique weight-loss program that's sweeping the nation! Dieting is a way of life for Donna, as she has accomplished something no other person on Earth has ever done before in the diet industry. She has recorded and counted her calories in her own diet journal for twenty-two years, something she doesn't expect the rest of the world to have to do. Donna's twenty-two years of obesity research led to the invention of the *net calorie*, which scientists across the country have deemed "the equation for thinness." Donna has discovered the most logical and innovative way of monitoring calories ever devised. She has combined the laws of chemistry, kinetics and thermodynamics and put them into a simple yet effective equation. The *net calorie* is a scientific breakthrough that takes dieting to a whole new level. Donna's matchless approach to weight loss has helped thousands of people lose weight. Some clients have lost over 100 pounds using her unprecedented method of dieting.

Donna leads you every step of the way down the path of weight loss. She turns the tables on conventional diets by exposing what actually goes on behind the scenes. This book discerns the difference between diet myth and diet truth. It teaches you how to become your own "diet detective" so that you can identify the factors that contributed to your own individual weight gain.

This book doesn't waste space on menus you won't follow and complicated recipes you'll never prepare. It gets right to the heart of the matter. This novel contains essential diet information that's never been revealed to the public. You can turn to any chapter and find beneficial diet advice. It's the world's first designer diet that shows you how to become your own diet coach. This book incorporates every facet of dieting by including a special section on how to help your family and friends lose weight. Donna understands that dieting is a family affair. She gets inside the mind of a dieter and provides unparalleled solutions to modify your behavior in order to achieve victorious weight loss. This book leaves no dietary stone unturned. It is the most complete guide to permanent weight loss ever written!

1. IN THE BEGINNING

Congratulations! You've purchased the book that will finally expose the truth about dieting. I've read hundreds of other diet books that make false promises and put unreasonable demands on you, and I find that the one common denominator about diets is that we are sick of being lied to. I invented this program because I discovered that the dieters have been over-counting their calories all these years. Once you learn the secrets of subtracting calories from your favorite foods, you'll discover how the truth will set you free to lose weight without feeling like you're dieting. Many diet authors have lied and distorted facts to appear authentic, taking you down the wrong path unknowingly.

I say these things because I speak from a lifelong experience of dieting. The best place to start is at the beginning so that you understand that this program was actually birthed out of necessity. When you're raised with an overweight family, you can choose two paths. The first is to eat like them and accept the fact that you're going to end up like the rest of the family. The second is to rebel and decide you are going to be a normal weight no matter how difficult the task may be.

I took the road less traveled and decided that I didn't want to endure the mental cruelty of being overweight. You may think this observation is a bit harsh at first glance, but if you could hear what my school friends and neighbors said about my overweight aunts, you would do just about anything to avoid obesity. It's not as if diets were anything new to me, because my aunts were always on some new diet. You always knew when they were about to embark upon the latest fad diet because they would boast and brag about their first week's weight loss. As a young child, it all seemed rather strange to me that the relatives who seemed to be dieting the most still weighed the most! The key word here is "seemed." I still remember the thought in my mind as if it were yesterday. I decided when I was twelve years old that I was going to show my family how to lose weight! I wanted to be an example for others to follow, and thus my dieting journey began. My first plan of action was to do the opposite of my overweight relatives.

I lived next door to my Italian grandparents until I was seventeen years old. My grandma was the designated family babysitter, so there were always children to be fed, which meant cooking and eating throughout the day. I was the oldest of the grandchildren and therefore was responsible for helping Grandma with the daily chores, which included cooking. I was exposed to more food choices in childhood than most people will see in a lifetime. My grandma was known for her culinary skills, and friends would gather at her house after school to enjoy her freshly baked desserts. The temptation was so unbearable that I decided to run for an hour every day after school so that I wouldn't be lured into eating. I figured the additional exercise would help me maintain my weight. Let me add that it wasn't easy to be athletic in a couch potato family. I was expecting my family to be proud of my endeavor, but instead I was discouraged from running. I'm from Syracuse, New York, so the weather is often a deterrent enough, but I was determined to be normal weight. I remember getting layers of clothing on and wrapping old bread bags around my feet so they wouldn't get wet and become numb. I would put oil on my face and then use a ski mask so that the bitter cold wouldn't build up ice on my face from my sweat and saliva. I would run no matter what the weather was and have done so in temperatures of twenty below zero. My family would say a harsh remark as I was going out the door, such as, "You could kill yourself if you slip on the ice and get run over by a car or a truck." But I'm a determined individual; therefore statements such as this only served to motivate me even more. The whole point here is to realize what extremes I was willing to go to in order to prevent obesity.

The workouts became more extreme as I grew older. I joined karate and starting lifting weights as well. If I gained weight, I would increase my level of exercise to make amends with myself. My schedule began to wear me down, but I continued in spite of my soreness. It's important to understand that I didn't consider myself a jock, because in fact my school nickname was "the brain." My first priority at that time in my life was to have the highest average possible in every class and to get a college scholarship, both of which I later achieved. The exercise was not something that I intended to excel in, even though I did. It was performed each day in order to avoid weight gain.

The next plan of action I devised was to eat less by eliminating breakfast and lunch. It was simple to cancel the first meal because that meant extra sleeping time in the morning. The second meal was eradicated by simply leaving my lunch in my locker and studying during lunch, or by selling my sandwich to a hungry student.

Soon it was time to stop punishing myself in order to evade my supposed obese destiny. This time I decided to use my head instead of my heart. My life had changed considerably, and with age comes wisdom, which was the prominent and contributing attribute to my diet discoveries. The first task was to research the current diet programs available and decide if they were worth giving a try. I then purchased and read over 100 different diet books. By then I had become a trained research scientist, and I realized that there were various discrepancies and multiple scientific blunders. It seemed as if there were no set standard that these books were based upon. If the authors continuously contradicted one another, how could the reader discern the truth? Your diet fate shouldn't depend upon which book you happen to purchase, but that's what can occur if you're not a perceptive dieter.

The next step was to decide which diet program I should embark upon. The only problem was, there wasn't one single diet I wanted to follow. Then I came up with a brilliant plan. I decided to rely upon science and develop my own program. Let's just say it's a diet jungle out there, and what I was about to invent was similar to blazing a new trail in the forest. If you've ever had to start a path where no man has gone before, or none that you know of in the last 50 years, then you understand the level of difficulty. You need to proceed slowly and have an eye for detail. You must discipline yourself to take small steps forward, because your next footstep could be into a snare of vines growing along the forest floor. It's easy to get tripped up and fall if you don't know where you're going. Therefore, you must proceed with caution and patience.

It's the same way for *you* on your weight loss journey. *You* are going to go down a new path this time, because the end of the road leads to a lifetime of freedom from obesity. The beauty of this expedition of weight loss is that I have already cleared the trail for you. After 20 years of research, the only logical diet that works for everyone is a program that allows you to become interactive and adjust the system according to your individual lifestyle. The diets that have specific menus and instruct you to obey their each and every command tend to ultimately destruct. When you're finished reading this book, you'll be able to discern the factors that contributed to your weight gain. Once you realize what caused the problem, then you can make the appropriate changes. The first rule you need to understand about successful dieting is that you're the one in charge. It's not up to an infomercial, a menu program, a pill, a particular food group, the combining of foods, or your family and friends. It's up to you to take responsibility for what you consume. Then once that's accomplished, you'll realize that *you're the boss of your weight loss.*

GENETIC PREDISPOSITION

One of the most devastating diet myths I can think of is the genetic predisposition toward obesity. It allows you to use the excuse that since your parents or siblings are overweight, you must be doomed to be obese as well. According to the laws of science, there are several proven genetic traits, and obesity isn't one of them. An example of a genetically inherited trait is the fact that every redhead that's born will have freckles. There is never an exception; if there were a single case, scientists would no longer deem it a genetic trait. Another genetic example they show you in seventh grade is that some of us can curl our tongues and some cannot; there is no in-between. Since there are many cases that disprove the genetic propensity to gain weight, you can get the thought out of your mind and not let it enter your weight loss equation.

A perfect example that disproves genetic weight gain comes from my own family. My aunt was married once and had no children; she then remarried a man who had one male child. My aunt was about 300 pounds when she married a thin man. Their eating habits were quite different. She would eat several large portions at dinner, and he was satisfied with one plate of food. After dinner, she would continue to munch upon cakes, cookies, candy, chips, and whatever food was available at the time. He on the other hand would drink beer or mixed drinks in lieu of food. She gained weight, and he stayed rather thin.

Their son was normal weight when he joined my family. His stepmother would now be the preparer of his breakfast, lunch, and dinner. I still remember him bringing two peanut butter and jelly sandwiches, grape juice, and a candy bar for lunch. He ate so many peanut butter sandwiches that the children nicknamed him Skippy, and he still has to deal with that nickname to this day. As soon as he started eating the food that his overweight stepmother prepared for him, he started to gain weight. He was starting to look like his stepmother, to whom he had no blood relation, instead of his thin father! This proves the point plainly and simply. If you are given too many calories as a child, you will gain weight.

The great news is you are not doomed to be overweight. Obesity is a learned behavior, because it is a result of poor eating habits. Your body has no choice but to gain weight when you take in more calories than you burn. The flip side of the whole situation is that we are gaining weight because of our eating habits, not our genetics. This can easily be reversed once you become a diet detective and see where the excess calories that don't add any volume to your diet are sneaking in. You are not programmed to be overweight. In fact, it is just the opposite. On a cellular replication basis, you are destined to live for 120 years! You are slated to be normal weight and live a healthy life!

GOING MOBILE

When I first started this diet company, I decided to do something that no other diet company had done in my whole region. I went to each client's home to give him or her a diet meeting. The reason I decided to have my diet meetings in my clients' residences is that I felt that weight loss is a family affair. I would then be able to study the influence each family member had on the dieter. This turned out to be quite an eye opener. This was done in order to study dieters in their own environment and to see the situations that each individual was dealing with. It gave me an opportunity to talk with family members and hear their side of the story. It also allowed me the liberty of looking into their refrigerators and cupboards to see what they were really eating. The experience was priceless. I've actually sat at a kitchen table with three generations of dieters and listened to each one discuss the reasons they were overweight. I visited their homes on a weekly basis, and they became more candid with us as time went on.

The diet program required each participant to be weighed and measured each week. It was amazing to see how many people were ashamed to weigh in, in front of their spouses and siblings. It was their choice whether to weigh themselves in front of the family or in private. The most enlightening part of the experience was how food affected their relationship with one another.

My first diet consultation on the road was back in 1985, and I only charged each client ten dollars per week. I put up a simple flyer on grocery store bulletin boards and in local gyms. The very first advertisement I designed read "Lose 10 pounds Quick." It had little tabs that you tore off with my company name and number. I went to check my signs to see how many people had torn off the phone number. Much to my surprise, the sign had already acquired graffiti. Written across the ad was "Just cut your head off." That put things into perspective. It was time to tell the consumer why my program was superior to all other diets. The best way I could do this was with scientific evidence and actual case studies. When I'm in your home, I can prove to the whole family that this diet is livable and successful.

I was anxiously anticipating my first diet meeting. I put on my business suit and arrived at the home. I was at the home ringing the doorbell, and there was no answer. There I was at my first meeting being stood up. As a last ditch effort, I decided to glance into the window. The curtain was drawn, and I saw a sight that would make a rookie diet counselor shudder. The two sisters who were about to join my program were sitting at the table with a large box of donuts in front of them. The larger sibling took the empty box of donuts, lifted the box to her mouth, and ate every last crumb that it contained. Thoughts began swirling around in my mind. If food is this important to them, how long will I be able to keep them away from those donuts? They were having what I call the "last supper," which is discussed in detail in the Getting Started chapter. The stark reality of teaching people how to lose weight was no easy chore. I was preparing myself mentally for the task.

I knocked and walked in, introduced myself, gave my diet pitch, and they both joined the program. The next part is usually the most difficult—the weighing and measuring. This usually upsets the dieter when they have to face the facts in writing. Every journey starts with the first step, however, and this step is the biggest one. They proceeded to weigh in. At this point a dieter can start to feel a sense of disgust as well as despair. This goes away after your second weigh-in and you see yourself losing weight and inches. (I've provided a weight and measurement chart in my Getting Started chapter. The sooner you use it, the quicker you will reach your goal.)

After they both were weighed and measured, I began to tell them their first week's instructions. (This is also provided in the Getting Started chapter.) But the moral of this story is that there's more to food than just eating it. If you haven't started a diet yet, then you have placed your love of food above the desire to be thin. When you think of weight loss, you assume that you will have to give up all of your favorite foods. If I thought that's what a diet was, I would procrastinate also! It was this issue that changed my whole outlook on dieting forever. I realized that a person could be given the world's most perfect eating plan, but it would be worthless to them if they didn't follow the program. How will they be able to follow a specific menu if they don't want to eat those exact foods? Then it hit me like a ton of bricks. It was like one of those old-fashioned cartoons when they show a character with a great idea and a light bulb goes off in his head. This wasn't just a light bulb; this was more like a light show! I knew that if I proceeded with my ingenious thought that it would be a difficult endeavor, but the results would far exceed the effort. So before I even walked in the door, I decided this was going to be a program like no other on Earth. I was secure in knowing that I could help everyone who was ready to diet to lose weight. Now you're probably wondering how I was going to accomplish such a goal. After all, you've heard false promises from plenty of diets. The answer is, it's not my diet. It's your diet. I tell every client at his or her first meeting, "I don't expect you to eat what I eat because it works for me. I want you to eat what you want and have it work for you!"

The most unusual aspect of this diet is frequently brought up at my client meetings. The dieters ask me, "How come you don't tell me exactly what to eat?" I do ask them to write down what they eat and become responsible for their actions, but I respond by telling them, "There are thousands of menu programs available, and you didn't follow them; why would mine be any different?" If I tell you what to eat, I am your diet mother, and then it puts you into what I call the "bad girl" or "good girl" syndrome. This is not the state of mind that results in changing your eating habits. This is a state of mind that sets you up for diet sabotage. You shouldn't think of "good" or "bad." Think of *change*.

2. CALCULATING YOUR NET CALORIES

THE DISCOVERY

Like most significant scientific advances, I invented the net calorie diet out of necessity. It all happened because of the introduction of the nutrition facts box. Before the onset of these facts, I would have to calculate the calories myself based upon the ingredients and their order of appearance on the label. For years, I've had to depend upon this method, which served me well, as I weigh less than 100 pounds at 5'2." Obviously, I was ciphering my calories correctly. You can imagine the anticipation I felt when I heard that the calories would now be made known publicly. I rushed right over to my favorite food emporium to see how I fared with the labels. Something was noticeably wrong from the start. My favorite whole-wheat pasta was listed as having the same calories as white enriched pasta. (I always say to my clients, "When God puts white wheat on Earth, I'll eat it. Until then I'll consume it the way it was intended.") It wouldn't take a food scientist to figure out that the whole-wheat version was better than the processed white one. Whole grains pass through the digestive tract much faster and helps to push the other food out along with it. Then I took a gander at white bread and my favorite dark whole-grain bread and noticed the same thing. How could white bread have fewer calories than brown bread? I decided to trust my caloric intuition, take action, and do the only logical thing: experiment.

THE CALORIE BURN

I've read numerous scientific documentation of the calorie burn, and there's one common factor these studies lack: confirmation of the theory on an actual human being. One day I was explaining net calories to a client, and I told her that the calorie burn theory works in a laboratory, but just look what happens if you drop a peanut in your oven. It turns brown and won't disintegrate. It will be there quite awhile. The longer it takes to burn, the more calories the product will appear to have. But the denser the product (more fibrous), the more difficult it will be to burn! The food appears to have higher calories when in fact only a fraction of it is absorbed in your body. I'm not saying that the calorie burn is totally incorrect; I'm stating that my digestive system is not that simple. I proved that if I were off by only 10 percent on my net calorie counting method, I would weigh 300 pounds by now! *What I've proven is that the only calories you need to count are the ones your body absorbs, not the ones it doesn't.*

THE JOURNEY OF THE CALORIE

The path that a food takes in the process of digestion determines the amount of calories that are available for absorption. The key factor here is to consume food that has a fast transit time in order to facilitate your weight loss. The dieter should use science to his or her advantage; the fewer calories absorbed, the less you weigh. The journey your calorie takes will determine the journey your weight takes. The good news is that you'll be eating more than you ever have before, and weighing less.

The way that the body digests food is different for each type of food that we eat. The total calories are derived from the carbohydrates, proteins, and fats. The body must distinguish between each type of food and process it according to its chemical composition. The net calories are the ones that you need to count, and the perfect examples are in corn and peas. If you look them up in a basic calorie counting book, they are both listed at 120 calories per cup and are the two highest-calorie vegetables. The reason for this is the calorie-counting method used to determine their caloric content. They both have a fiber-like outer lining that takes time to burn. The longer it takes the food to burn, the higher the traditional calorie count, so the logical conclusion for corn and peas is that you shouldn't have to count the calories that pass through the body undigested.

The reason fruits and vegetables are a dieter's ally is because of the journey they take in the body after they are ingested raw. In addition, they are mainly comprised of distilled water, so they provide a feeling of fullness. They are heavy by weight yet low in calories. This fills up the stomach. The stomach is like a combination of a juicer and an acid bath. The food empties into it, and the stomach tries to break it down. The body takes time to digest food that has fiber. This process therefore keeps the dieter satisfied longer.

The fiber in the food is then transported down the digestive tract, taking calories along with it. The magnificent part of fiber is its ability to absorb water. This accomplishes an important goal for the dieter, which is a feeling of fullness without consuming more calories. The key to success with any diet is to be

Then complete the calculation:

Net Calories = 90–28

Net Calories = 62

It's even simpler to calculate your net calories based upon your specific food selections. The best choices are the items that have the highest fiber content or are raw. These products have a lower net calorie value, which means that you'll be able to consume a higher-volume diet. The optimum method of determining your net caloric intake is to utilize the charts. You simply look up the calorie with its corresponding fiber value to find the net calories. They are divided into common caloric increments for ease of use. Most of my clients perform the math in their head as they are shopping so that they can purchase the food with the lowest net calories.

It is important to remember that if you eat more than the portion size on the label, then you must adjust the calories and fiber according to the portion you consumed. If for instance you eat two portions, then double the calories in order to determine the appropriate net calories.

PASTA: THE DIETER'S BEST FRIEND

The net calorie is similar to the English language because they both have exceptions to the rule. Many examples can be found in the food charts, but I want to highlight one of them now: pasta. I've chosen pasta to represent the first exception to the PAR rule for several reasons. First, it's a dieter's best friend because it provides ample volume for satisfaction while dieting. The second rationale for using pasta as the premiere example is that it's so versatile that you can prepare it several times a week without having the same taste or flavor.

The reason why pasta is an exception is that the calories on the label are listed for dry pasta. Since we eat our pasta cooked, the actual calorie content must be adjusted to account for the part of the grain that remains in the boiling water. There are several calorie-counting books that list the value of cooked pasta as approximately 150 calories per cup cooked, which comes from a 2-ounce serving (dry), depending on the shape of the pasta. However, this caloric value does not take into account the unabsorbed calories due to its fiber content.

The above value is for white enriched pasta, which contains 2 g of fiber per serving; therefore, its only 138 net calories per cup. That's great news for a dieter because the net calories are even less for whole-wheat pasta due to its high fiber content. Since pasta ranges in fiber from 2 grams for white pasta to 10 grams for whole wheat flax pasta, the differences in net calories are listed below for your convenience.

PASTA: NET CALORIES (COOKED)

Fiber (g) Per cup	Net calories per ½ cup	Net calories per cup	Net calories per 4 cups	Net calories per 8 cups
2	69	138	552	1104
3	66	132	528	1056
4	63	126	504	1008
5	60	120	480	960
6	57	114	456	912
7	54	108	432	864
8	51	102	408	816
9	48	96	384	768
10	45	90	360	720

3. EASY NET CALORIE CHARTS

Use these charts to look up your net calories the easy way. All the calculations have been done for you. Just locate your calorie and fiber values, and the chart tells you the corresponding net calories, most of which are for cooked foods.

50 calories		60 Calories	
Fiber	Net Calories	Fiber	Net Calories
1	44	1	54
2	38	2	48
3	32	3	42
4	26	4	36
5	20	5	30
6	14	6	24
		7	18
70 Calories		80 Calories	
Fiber	Net Calories	Fiber	Net Calories
1	64	1	74
2	58	2	68
3	52	3	62
4	46	4	56
5	40	5	50
6	34	6	44
7	28	7	38
90 Calories		100 Calories	
Fiber	Net Calories	Fiber	Net Calories
1	84	1	94
2	78	2	88
3	72	3	82
4	66	4	76
5	60	5	70

6	54	6	64
7	48	7	58
8	42	8	52
200 Calories		**300 Calories**	
Fiber	**Net Calories**	**Fiber**	**Net Calories**
1	194	1	294
2	188	2	288
3	182	3	282
4	176	4	276
5	170	5	270
6	164	6	264
7	158	7	258
8	152	8	252
9	146	9	246
10	140	10	240
11	134	11	234
12	128	12	228
13	122	13	222
14	116	14	216
15	110	15	210

NET CALORIES FOR COMMON FOODS

Note: Many of these figures are exceptions to the rule due to being raw, and some are rounded off for easier counting.

FRUIT

Apple	1 w/skin	50	Lemon	1	5
Apricots	2	25	Lime	1	5
Banana	1 med.	50	Mandarin orange	1	50
Berries (all)	1 C.	50	Mango	1/2	50
Blackberries	1 C.	50	Nectarine	1	40
Boysenberries	1 C.	50	Orange	1	40
Blueberries	1 C.	50	Papaya	1 C.	35

Cantaloupe	1 C.	40	Peach	1 med.	25
Cherries	15	40	Pear	1 med.	50
Dates	1	15	Persimmon	1	25
Elderberries	1 C.	50	Pineapple	1 C.	50
Figs	1	25	Plum	1	20
Grapefruit	1	50	Pomegranate	1	50
Grapes	1 C.	40	Raspberries	1 C.	50
Guava	1	25	Strawberries	1 C.	50
Honeydew	1 C.	50	Tangerine	1	25
Kiwi	1	30	Watermelon	1 C.	30

VEGETABLES

Alfalfa sprouts	1 C.	2	Peas, sugar snap	1 C.	30
Artichoke	1 C.	50	Peppers	1 C.	14
Asparagus	1 C.	30	Potato	1 C.	110
Avocado	1	150	Potato, sweet	1 C.	130
Bamboo shoots	1 C.	30	Pumpkin	1 C.	35
Beets	1 C.	30	Radish	1 C.	5
Broccoli	1 C.	20	Rhubarb	1 C.	40
Brussels sprouts	1 C.	40	Rutabaga	1 C.	40
Cabbage, all	1 C.	5	Sauerkraut	1 C.	20
Carrots	1 C.	30	Seaweed	1 C.	35
Cauliflower	1 C.	15	Shallots	1 C.	5
Celery	1 C.	2	Spinach	1 C.	5
Corn	1 C.	60	Squash, zucchini	1 C.	10
Cucumbers	1 C.	10	Squash, winter		
Eggplant	1 C.	15	Acorn	1 C.	80
Green beans	1 C.	30	Butternut	1 C.	55
Greens, steamed	1 C.	15	Hubbard	1 C.	70
Kale	1 C.	5	Spaghetti	1 C.	30
Lettuce	1 C.	5	Succotash	1 C.	100
Mushrooms	1 C.	14	Swamp cabbage	1 C.	5
Okra	1 C.	27	Tomato	1 C.	20
Onions	1 C.	40	Turnip	1 C.	20
Parsnips	1 C.	80	Turnip greens	1 C.	2

Peas, green	1 C.	60		Water chestnuts	1 C.	50
Peas, snow pea	1 C.	30		Yam	1 C.	70

BEANS

Adzuki	1 C.	175		Lentil	1 C.	110
Baked w/o sugar	1 C.	120		Lima	1 C.	130
Black (boiled)	1 C.	135		Mung	1 C.	120
Black turtle	1 C.	145		Navy	1 C.	150
Broad beans	1 C.	100		Pinto	1 C.	130
Butter beans	1 C.	120		Red	1 C.	120
Cannelloni	1 C.	100		Refried	1 C.	160
Chickpeas	1 C.	150		Soybeans	1 C.	120
Cowpeas	1 C.	120		Wax	1 C.	30
Fava	1 C.	120		White	1 C.	150
Great northern	1 C.	120		Yard long	1 C.	120
Kidney	1 C.	130		Yellow	1 C.	140

GRAINS

Barley (cooked)	1 C.	120		Rice flour, white	1 C.	450
Buckwheat flour	1 C.	225		Rye flour, dark	1 C.	250
Carob flour	1 C.	100		Rye flour, light	1 C.	275
Corn germ	1 C.	100		Soybean flour	1 C.	250
Corn flour	1 C.	260		Soy flour, defatted	1 C.	200
Corn meal	1 C.	250		Wheat bran	1 C.	50
Millet, cooked	1 C.	175		Wheat flour, enrich	1 C.	450
Oat bran	1 C.	150		Wheat flour, whole	1 C.	250
Potato flour	1 C.	500		Wheat germ, toasted	1 C.	225
Rice bran	1 C.	150		Wheat germ, raw	1 C.	150
Rice flour, brown	1 C.	250				

There are more net calorie charts in the appendix.

4. YOUR DIET COACH

When my clients begin this program, I ask them who they share their meals with, because those people influence the outcome of the diet. Do the social situations in your life lead to overeating, or is there a particular person who causes you to overeat? Will your spouse and children help or hinder your weight loss? I've had plenty of dieters tell me that their spouse brought home their favorite pastry to enjoy after dinner, knowing they were on a diet. If your spouse knew you shouldn't have them, they're not being a good diet coach. It's like bringing home a pack of cigarettes to your wife who just quit smoking!

In order to achieve long-term weight loss, you should be honest with the people you dine with and tell them you're serious about dieting. Why wouldn't you? Is it because of a fear of failure or the dread of being ridiculed? Some friends or family say things like, "Oh, not another diet!" "How much money did you spend this time?" Or "Diets never work for you." It's time to make it perfectly clear to them that you truly desire to reach your weight loss goal and would appreciate their help!

The whole family should be interactive with this diet and eat the recipes together. After all, nutritious eating habits need to start when you are young. Families come together in a time of crisis, so why not use this diet as a way of bringing your family closer together? *When you tell them the truth, all things work out for the better.* Let them know you need their support. Chances are there are some people in your family who could stand to lose a couple of pounds, so why not ask them to diet with you? After all, there is strength in numbers.

You are more apt to lose weight when you have a diet coach. *I always tell my clients that there are plenty of excellent athletes, but the greatest ones have one thing in common: an even greater coach.* One of my all-time favorite coaches, Vince Lombardi, stated, "It's not how many times you fall that counts; it's how many times you get back up." I think of his words when I'm competing athletically, and it urges me on to win!

A MESSAGE TO THE DIET COACH
(A SIGNIFICANT OTHER'S GUIDE TO BECOMING A DIET COACH)

"Honey, I started a diet today." What's the first thought that comes to mind when your partner utters the four-letter word "diet"? It usually brings forth several subconscious reactions like, "I hope she doesn't get into one of her moods because she can't eat everything she wants to." Or "I wonder if we'll have to live on rabbit food for the next two weeks." Your defense mechanisms are a result of your experiences with past diets. Most short-term weight loss schemes don't live up to their promises. It's therefore logical to understand why you're skeptical when your loved one embarks on a diet program. It's almost as if you expect her to fail, because every time she's dieted previously, the weight came back. It's time to forget the past and celebrate the fact that your partner is now on a program that teaches her how to adapt a diet to her individual lifestyle.

Here are three basic scenarios that can occur when someone begins a diet.

FIRST SCENARIO
ONE PERSON IS DIETING AND LIVING WITH A NORMAL WEIGHT PARTNER.

This particular situation presents several obstacles for the dieter, which can be conquered when you, the non-dieting partner, take on the role of the diet coach. Following the scenarios are some adjustments that you should adopt to help your beloved accomplish a weight loss goal.

SECOND SCENARIO
BOTH PARTNERS ARE OVERWEIGHT, AND ONLY ONE OF THEM GOES ON A DIET.

This can be a volatile situation, because the partner who is not on the diet can become angry or jealous of the dieting partner. The real issue is that one person is on the diet and the other isn't ready to diet at the present time. If you're the overweight partner who's not dieting, it's important not to sabotage your loved one's decision. There are rules below for diet coaches, and they may even help both of you get on the road to weight loss together.

You may not be ready to diet because you've never been on a program worth staying on. It's time to expand your horizons and give yourself a chance to experience what this book can do to change the way you feel about dieting forever!

If you aren't mentally prepared to start a diet just because your partner begins a weight loss program, then you still have an obligation to help him or her to achieve a goal. You know deep down inside that you really should be losing weight, but you need some motivation. You couldn't ask for more inspiration than living with a dieter. If you really want to benefit from their endeavors, then let them pave the way for you. If your loved one wants to make a delicious diet casserole for dinner, then sit and enjoy the meal. You'll probably end up losing a few pounds, and this may provide ample encouragement to start dieting yourself. When we see others succeed, the desire to do the same is quite contagious.

THIRD SCENARIO
BOTH PARTNERS ARE OVERWEIGHT, AND THEY START A WEIGHT LOSS PROGRAM TOGETHER.

This seems like the perfect situation because the couple can operate as a team. The one major setback that can occur in this situation is when one member of the team decides to binge and in turn convinces their partner to do the same. Then before you know it, the whole concept of dieting is a thing of the past, or something you'll try later on. The optimum way to avoid this pitfall is to have the most disciplined partner declared the Diet Captain. The Diet Captain's duty is to prevent mutiny on the bounty. This is when the weaker partner tries to convince you to cheat on your diet. It's your job to curtail the thought before it becomes an action. This is best accomplished by reminding your partner that the binge will only result in feelings of remorse and guilt, which are counterproductive to weight loss. It only takes ten minutes to consume thousands of calories, so why not let the time pass and think about the consequences before you do the damage? You should both discuss the outcome of the binge together. Then remind your partner of the importance of losing weight. If he or she still feels an uncontrollable urge to binge, then each of you should write down the top five reasons why you want to lose weight and discuss them together. Then it's time to try some low-calorie substitution recipes instead of the food you intend to binge upon. This will enable you to satisfy your urges and stay within their caloric limits at the same time. Since each of you will be a coach, you both need to read the rules below.

BASIC RULES FOR THE DIET COACH

1. Don't tempt your loved one by purchasing food gifts like chocolates, cake, candy, cookies, and other high-calorie desserts.

2. If you absolutely must eat forbidden foods, then do so at work or in privacy, not in front of your diet partner.

3. It's important to be sincerely enthusiastic and supportive while your partner is dieting.

4. Don't remind the dieter of any past dieting experiences that didn't pan out as planned.

5. If you regularly eat out, it's best to go to a restaurant that offers low-calorie fare, or avoid the trip altogether and visit a museum or art gallery instead.

6. If your family has take-out traditions or home deliveries that include high-calorie meals, put down the phone and prepare a romantic gourmet diet meal together instead.

7. In order to show you're in the dieter's court, offer to become involved in the particulars of the diet.

8. To promote exercise while dieting, join a fitness center with your partner or take up a new sport you can enjoy together or go for a daily walk.

9. If your dieting partner won't divulge his or her weight, it's about time you both faced reality and worked together toward achieving the goal. It's not the particular number on the scale that really matters; what's important is that the number is getting lower. Once the truth is out about their actual body weight, the burden of carrying around a secret will be lifted from their shoulders, allowing you as the dieting partner to establish a bond of trust. When a dieting loved one confides in you, it's a golden opportunity because you can get a true sense of their situation.

10. If your diet partner strays from the diet and binges, don't use it as an excuse to ridicule or insult them just because of their lapse in dietary discipline. I'm sure that you've had setbacks in life, and it doesn't help when your loved ones remind you of your mistakes or moments of weakness. The best thing to do in this situation is to forget about the cheating episode and encourage them to start the diet program again as soon as possible. This is a perfect time to offer compliments in regard to the dietary progress they have accomplished so far. It's always a good idea to mention that you've

noticed that your diet partner is losing weight, and let them know how much you appreciate it.

DIET BUDDIES, FOES, AND TRAITORS

DIET BUDDIES

There are three main types of people whom you will encounter when you embark on your weight loss endeavor. The first is the most obvious. When you start to diet, it's quite simple to recognize who your diet buddies are. These are the friends, family, and co-workers who fully support your decision. They're the people who remind you that you're dieting when you reach for that chocolate-covered donut at break time. They casually walk by with a remark like, "Aren't you supposed to be on a diet?" At that point you start to wonder if they're a friend or foe and whether you should have told them you were on a diet to begin with. They represent your diet conscience. When you're following the program, you love them, but when you want to cheat, you loathe them. When you start to lose a few pounds, they're the friends that tell you, "You look like you lost weight." They ask you what diet you are on, and all of a sudden, they're willing to take dietary advice from you. You need to use their support and incentive in a positive manner.

If a person in your life is willing to go beyond being a diet buddy and support you as your diet coach, let them. Verbal encouragement is so important to your success. If you don't have a diet coach, then you should acquire one. If you're married, the first choice should be your spouse. After all, they reap the benefits immediately. They get to admire your new slim and trim physique. A husband and wife team is a dynamic duo when they help each other diet. The perfect example is Jack LaLanne and his wife. They still look wonderful and are very attracted to each other after all these years. I can't help but think how many relationships will be saved and rejuvenated when overweight spouses become normal weight spouses. I'm not advocating divorce on the grounds of obesity, but it still happens. I feel that it's a responsibility to your loved one to maintain a normal weight so that you can enjoy many healthy and romantic years together. Plainly and simply, obesity reduces your lifespan!

The first objective of your diet coach is to eat only the foods you can have when they're with you. I tell my clients that if their spouse sits there with a bag of chips and dip while they're watching a movie together, he doesn't really expect you to nibble on carrot sticks the whole time, does he? Don't lead your spouse into temptation. If you absolutely must eat high-calorie food, then do so while you're alone. When you eat forbidden food in front of a dieter, you automatically condone the action. It makes a statement that cries out, "Hey, I'm going to have this food; wouldn't you like to be able to eat some of it?" You then start to justify the action by telling yourself that having just a little bit won't hurt. "I can always go back on my diet tomorrow."

The only logical solution is to eat the same foods together. A diet is technically a nutritious method of eating in order to sustain a healthy lifestyle, and that should make it compatible with everyone. If you're a dieter, but your spouse is not overweight, you can simply serve them a larger portion of the meal. It's important that you continue with your standard operating procedures. You shouldn't have to feel left out or cheated at dinner just because you're on a diet. Don't sit there with a diet meal and prepare the family high-calorie cuisine. I have always told my clients that if you don't start feeding your children lower-calorie food, I'll see them on the diet in about ten years! Dieting is a family affair, and it should benefit your whole family. You will learn to adopt lower calorie cooking options that taste great and provide abundant volume.

It's time to call the household together for a meeting. First, tell your spouse and children you intend to succeed. Next, ask them not to tempt you by eating forbidden food in front of you. Then give them an opportunity to provide support. Let them help out in the kitchen and prepare gourmet diet meals as a project. Some of my most poignant memories of my loved ones take place in the kitchen. It's a perfect opportunity to use the diet to bring the family together in order to achieve a common goal: eating healthier food in order to live a longer life. (See also the diet coach rules in this book.)

DIET FOES

The second type of person you come across is the diet foe. It seems like every time you try to lose weight, they feel a need to sabotage your diet. The typical diet enemies are the people who want to order out every Friday because it's payday or it's the weekend, so let's celebrate! You try to restrain yourself from cheating, yet these characters still provoke you! You tell them, "I don't really need to order a sub. I've already brought a salad and fruit for lunch, so no thank you!" They in turn ridicule you until you feel like a jerk if you don't join the eating spree. It puts you in a situation where you feel less pressure if you just give in and say yes rather than explain that you're dieting and that their food choices are too high in calories for you to consume. The decision here will set precedent. If you allow other people to convince you to overeat, they will continue to do so. You need to take a stand and let them know that you will not allow other people to influence what you can or can't eat. Peer pressure is a powerful force. It's something we always preach to our children, so then what right do we have to give into it ourselves. It is a perfect time to show by example that dieters have willpower.

The strange thing about the whole situation is that the diet foes are usually overweight. They might be jealous of you because you're losing weight. Perhaps they want you to binge so that they aren't the only ones who look bad. After all, misery loves company. If you're in a room with overweight people who are eating, and you're the only dieter, be on guard. It's like having a bleeding cut and swimming in the ocean with a group of sharks. They're waiting to attack, so to speak. You represent a diet to them. You are a reminder of something they should be doing. The way that you overcome this situation is to stand firm on your decision to diet.

DIET TRAITORS

The third type of person you meet is the diet traitor. This is not as obvious as it seems. It all begins when two people join forces in order to beat the battle of the bulge. It all starts out on a good note, and somehow it ends up going out of tune. The old adage that two heads are better than one doesn't always apply to diets. I'll give you a perfect real life example. I had two lifelong friends join my program together. They came to their diet meetings at the same time and even worked together. One was the school secretary and the other a teacher. They could therefore bolster each other's confidence on a daily basis. This is a perfect case scenario as long as they're both dieting. They were off to a great start and used each other as coaches. Then one of them decided to go off the program. That person is then by dietary definition the diet traitor. This traitor convinces the diet buddy to go off the program in order to justify his or her own actions. They either both lost weight or gained weight. It's great to have support and motivation, but it shouldn't determine your individual weight loss. If your diet friend tries to become a diet traitor, don't let that person drag you down as well. It's much easier to quit a diet than it is to stay on one.

You should tell your diet partner that your weight loss goal is important and you will not be a part of their overeating lifestyle anymore. Instead of letting them persuade you to cheat, why not convince them to stay on the diet? If they decide they're not going to diet now, then find activities that you can share with them that don't involve food or binging. It's time to be a good example and show them that your diligence is paying off. Once they see you lose weight, they will either start their diet again or grow envious of your success. Regardless of what happens to them, you have to remember you're dieting for yourself, not to please them. Don't let anyone change your mind. You shouldn't let peer pressure enter into the picture. Your weight loss should not depend upon whether your friend is on a diet. If you really enjoy dieting with a partner, then find a new diet buddy—one who will help you lose weight, not gain weight.

You can't let your friends, family, and co-workers determine how or what you eat. If they're overweight, chances are you'll find yourself eating forbidden food with them because they condone the action. Everyone likes to think that they eat well, but if they really did, they wouldn't be overweight. People who are not dieting don't like to be told what they can and cannot eat. No one wants to hear a diet lecture from a skinny person when they're overweight. People eat what they really want to eat, and they make excuses in order to do so. This is the exact reason you're dieting now. You've eaten too many calories in the past and must reduce your caloric intake in order to lose weight. If you eat what an overweight person eats, you'll weigh what an overweight person weighs. It's time to take responsibility for your own actions, and don't fret about what other people eat. You have to live with your body; they do not. It's important to think of your future and visualize the benefits that you'll receive when you lose weight.

THE 60/40 DEAL

If this were offered to me in a partnership, I would have to decline. The 60/40 agreement I'm referring to is not the distribution of business profits. It's the percentage of calories consumed by a dieter (40 percent) compared to their spouse or significant other (60 percent). The key word here is *calories*, which means that you won't have to compromise volume, so you still get to feel full, and the trade off yields weight loss.

It's a common mistake to think that you should be able to eat as much as your spouse. I've heard numerous complaints from my female clients regarding how much their husbands can eat without gaining as much weight as they do. Then I ask them a key question: how much does your spouse weigh? The reply is always as I was expecting. They will state that he weighs much more than they do and is about a foot taller. For discussion purposes, the most typical case scenario is the 5'3" wife weighing in at 150 pounds and the 6'2" husband who weighs 200 pounds. The wife in this situation is gaining weight as the years go by because eating too many calories will eventually catch up with anybody. If you consume the same amount of calories as a 200-pound person, you may eventually weigh 200 pounds.

The way we serve food is a learned behavior that's generally passed down from one generation to the next. It's such an automatic routine that you don't really think about the portion size; you just serve the food equally. When you cook a roast, you slice the meat symmetrically and serve it so everyone receives their fair share of the meat. The way we distribute our food determines how the calories are allotted to each person, and a dieter doesn't want to share calories equally with a non-dieter. A dieter just wants to feel full and satisfied. It's important to understand that you won't be sacrificing volume, which is the key to staying satisfied both mentally and physically while dieting.

Here's an example of the 60/40 deal. If you're serving hamburgers, baked potatoes, and green beans for dinner, the concept is to distribute the high-calorie items sparingly to yourself and expand the volume of your meal with the lower calorie foods.

Let's take a closer look at how this deal works to benefit you and promote weight loss on a daily basis. Let's start by calculating the calories of the meal that you serve to your spouse.

Non Dieter's Dinner		
Food	**Portion**	**NET Calories**
Hamburger Roll	1	150
Hamburger	6 oz.	480
Cheese	1 sl.	100
Ketchup	2 Tbsp.	30
Mayonnaise	2 Tbsp.	200
Pickle slices	4	5
Baked Potato	1 large	200
Butter	2 Tbsp.	200
Sour Cream	1 Tbsp.	30
Green Beans	1 C.	30
Soda	1 reg.	150
		1,575 calories

As innocent as the meal seems, it's obvious that when you calculate the calories in this dinner, it has far too many to consume while dieting. So be sure to reduce the calories and increase the volume for the dieting partner's portion.

Dieter's Dinner		
Food	**Portion**	**NET Calories**
Whole Grain Roll	1	100
Or		
Diet Bread	2	
Hamburger	3½ oz.	280
Low-Calorie Cheese	1 sl.	50
Lettuce	1 C.	5
Tomato slices	4	2
Onion slices	4	2
Pickle slices	4	5
Baked Potato	1 large	200
Butter Sprinkles	1 Tbsp.	5
Low Calorie Sour Cream	2 Tbsp.	39
Green Beans	2 C.	60
Diet Soda	1	0
		748 calories

Now it's time to do the diet math. The total calories of the two meals are 2,323 calories. The amount that the dieter consumed is 32 percent. This is actually better than the 60/40 rule allows for sharing a meal with someone that weighs more than you.

The ideal way to approach the 60/40 deal is to categorize food according to its caloric density. The foods that contain 100 or more calories per ounce should be consumed sparingly because the calories tend to add up much too quickly. Foods in this group are generally meats, sweets, and oil. The most calorically dense foods are fats. The edibles that contain the lowest caloric density are fruits and vegetables, which are a dieter's best friends because they can increase the volume of your meals. The above example illustrates the use of adding extra veggies to your dinner in order to reduce the calories and simultaneously increase the volume.

The trick to adhering to the 60/40 deal is to break the rules of how you typically serve your meal. You need to alter the mindset that demands the right to consume as many calories as your spouse or eating partner. For example, if you order an eight-slice pizza, the natural way of distribution is to put equal pieces on each plate and then begin eating. This is one reason why a pizza should be ordered unsliced, so that the dieter can determine the size of each slice. The dieter's way of ordering a pizza and eating the pie is discussed in the chapter entitled Breaking the Rules.

Once you overcome the food equality dilemma, you'll be able to eat your meal without feeling cheated. The whole concept of being able to eat as many calories as someone who weighs more than you is mathematically unsound. When you take the time to think it through logically, you'll understand that this line of reasoning results in weight gain. It therefore should be altered in order to promote weight loss. The great news is that you won't be decreasing your portion; you'll actually be increasing the amount of food you consume when you apply the 60/40 deal properly!

5. GETTING STARTED

This is the day you start your diet. It is the moment you've been waiting for, or perhaps the day you've been avoiding for years. It may be the day after New Year's or a Monday, but either way there is never a better time to start a diet than today. The first thing you need to do is to prepare yourself mentally and get in the mode of dieting. Then make a commitment to yourself that this is an important goal in your life. Don't set time and weight-loss goals that are impossible to achieve—like trying to lose 20 pounds in two weeks—and then quit if you don't. The first week of dieting should be an easy one, not a starvation plan.

Now is the time to weigh in. If you're dreading this moment, it's time to turn over a new dietary leaf. There are several reasons why you should weigh yourself the day you start dieting. The first rationale for doing so is that it's imperative that you give yourself the opportunity to succeed. If you don't step on the scale initially, then you'll be depriving yourself of an accomplishment that you don't even know you've achieved. It's important that you understand that not weighing in is like sabotaging your diet before you start it. The second intent for weighing yourself is that it provides future motivation to stay on the program. I've had diet clients whom I had to prod to the scale, and they were upset at the moment. Then when they came back the next week, they were glowing and grinning ear to ear as they boasted of their 7-pound weight loss. This was a turning point in their lives, as it shall be in yours also. You owe it to yourself to reap the benefits of your dieting endeavor from the moment you start it.

WEIGHT AND MEASUREMENT CHART

Date	Weight	Chest	Waist	Hips	Arms	Thighs	Calf	Inch Loss	Weight Loss

MODE OF DIETING

The most important factor in the equation of weight loss is your frame of mind. As you're reading this book, have you decided that you'll wait until next Monday to start the program? This is a perfect example of your state of mind. The other case in point is the special occasion dieter. When a client comes to me and says that he needs to lose weight for a wedding, a cruise, or a class reunion he will be attending, the success rate is phenomenal! This only proves my point about your mindset. When you're really determined to lose weight and there is a sense of urgency, you do it. If the diet can wait until next week, then it will.

The process of dieting starts in your mind, so you need to prepare yourself mentally to diet. The battle of the bulge is won by the brain, not the body. You're in control; so don't let anything get in the way of your goal. I still don't know why dieters say they're either on or off a diet. Don't put yourself in this frame of mind; remember that the word diet means an *ongoing* way of eating.

The most important thing you must do to achieve success on my diet is be accountable for what you eat. Once you face the facts, you can plan your strategy. You will be able to live on this program because it is designed by you, for you.

The problem with waiting to diet is what you consume prior to your diet. If you gain 2–4 pounds on a pre-diet binge, then your first week might not result in weight loss. The worst-case scenario is stepping on the scale after a week of serious dieting and seeing that your weight remained the same.

THE LAST SUPPER

The final cheating episode before you start a diet is what I call the Last Supper. For twenty years I've been listening to excuses like "I'm entitled to it" and "I deserve it" and "I'll be giving up my favorite foods and eating rabbit food, so why not have one last meal that I'm not held responsible for?" First of all, this type of dieting mentally sets you up for failure. When a person categorizes food like this, it prompts the mind instead of the body. Don't have it in your mind that "diet" food is tasteless, boring, and consists of difficult to prepare recipes! If you thought you could eat several plates of generously portioned pasta with cheese and meatballs and still lose weight, you would eat it, wouldn't you? Many dieters ask, "Do I have to cook in order to lose weight?" No, but you deserve it, plus my recipes take less time to prepare than it takes to polish your nails.

Secondly, the last supper will add some weight to the old scale and tip the weights against you, which causes a time delayed weight gain. The final binge day can add up to 5,000 or more calories, yet you wonder, *What's the harm in that? I'm going to starve myself the next day.* Here's what happens to your body. The exact time it takes to gain weight when excess calories are consumed is not a perfect science. It depends on multiple co-factors such as metabolism, transit time, fiber content, and water in the system. Therefore you could gain weight from your binge 3 or 4 days after your initial weigh-in (starting weight). So the case scenario is this: you weigh in after you diet for a week, and all of a sudden, you've gained a pound, and there goes the motivation right out the door. Already your defense mechanism starts to rear its ugly head. "Well that diet didn't work! Why bother?" The fact is you gained 3 pounds from your pre-diet eating spree and lost 2 pounds dieting, and it doesn't take a rocket scientist to figure out the math. Now after a week of dieting, you look like you gained weight when in fact you lost weight. The moral of the story is, don't have too many last suppers!

THE PERFECT DIETER

The way you proceed to diet in the very beginning will determine whether you stay on the program. Here are some examples of actual diet clients. I called these people the "perfect dieters." I warned them against it, and they didn't seem to listen. The perfect dieter starts out his week with the lowest caloric intake he can tolerate. Basically, he starves himself in order to expedite his weight loss. He then proceeds to work out as much as the average athlete in order to get to his goal weight even sooner. Now you ask, "What's wrong with this client? They appear to be doing all the right things." The problem with this behavior is that it restricts their food intake so drastically that they can't wait to quit so that they can eat all the foods that they've given up. I've seen clients lose 10 pounds in one week and then quit. That sounds crazy, but this happens because the dieter set unreasonable goals and went on a diet that wasn't livable.

Don't make a diet so difficult to follow that you stop and then tell your family and friends that the program was too restrictive. There is no such thing to me as quitting a diet. There are just days when you eat more calories than others. Many clients ask me, "How long will it take me to lose 20 pounds, because I have a wedding to attend in 2 weeks?"

Realistically you can lose about 3–4 pounds per week, of which 2–3 pounds are fat loss, therefore you must allow yourself time to achieve your weight-loss goal. *Set achievable, not unbelievable goals!*

ME AND MY METABOLISM

It's the latest dietary craze. You can't turn a page in a women's or health magazine without seeing an advertisement that promises to boost your metabolism and melt the pounds away. The promises are so outrageous that you have to chuckle or else cry at the thought of how many innocent citizens have purchased these overpriced products. I recently saw a magazine with a cover stating they were about to divulge the 30 foods that increase your metabolism. I turned to the appropriate page and found 15 vegetables and 15 fruits. Surprise, surprise, surprise. There are hundreds of products that falsely claim to be metabolic miracle pills. Who do you trust and where do you turn to? I have told my clients that science is proven. It doesn't require trust or faith; it presents the facts and then you are armed with the knowledge to make a logical decision. Most companies rely on testimony to push their products. This is the absolute worst-case scenario because it is anecdotal. In a court of law, this wouldn't even be considered evidence; it would be automatically dismissed as hearsay! This means the statement must be stricken from the court records and disregarded.

The first thing a dieter must do is determine how many net calories she can consume in order to maintain her weight. Plenty of dieters run around telling the rest of the world that they are unable to lose weight because they have a slow metabolism. Yet they have never kept track of how many calories they consume, not one day of their life. The reason I developed this diet is because I truly eat fewer calories than anyone I have ever met or studied in order to sustain my weight. If there's such a thing as a slow metabolism, I would be the perfect example. The uncanny thing about the metabolism is that the average dieter wants to complain about it as an excuse to be overweight. If you actually have a problem, then deal with it and work toward solving it. If for instance you find out after an eye exam that you can't see far away, you don't keep asking other people to describe other objects and read the road signs for you. No, instead you go to the eyeglass store and purchase the appropriate glasses. You need to first determine where your individual metabolism is at.

THE GREAT METABOLISM TEST

You are about to embark upon the most enlightening journey of your life. The adventure starts when you realize that your body is not programmed to gain weight. Your first step is to take the great metabolism test.

A good way to rate your metabolism is to find out how many calories it takes to maintain your current weight. For instance, suppose you find that you must eat 2,000 net calories a day just to maintain your existing weight. This tells you that any daily diet with less than 2,000 net calories should therefore produce weight loss. You no longer need to suffer through painful diets of a measly 800 net calories per day, because you're now aware that you can eat 1,600 net calories a day and still lose weight! A diet shouldn't mean starvation and depravation. It should mean satisfaction and gratification!

Therefore, you need to have an accurate evaluation of your caloric intake while you're not dieting if you want to know how much you can lose. Most people haven't got a clue as to how many calories they actually consume in one day. This diet will be a lesson for life. One method is to write down everything you eat and drink for 7 days and add up the calories and calculate your average caloric intake. Simply add up your calories from each day and divide your total weekly calories by 7 to determine your daily average caloric intake (ACI).

The following is an actual example of how to compute your ACI:

Monday	Day 1: 2,523 cal
Tuesday	Day 2: 2,824 cal
Wednesday	Day 3: 2,405 cal
Thursday	Day 4: 2,708 cal
Friday	Day 5: 2,852 cal
Saturday	Day 6: 2,973 cal
Sunday	Day 7: 3,027 cal.
	Total Calories = 19,312

Total Calories = 19,312

Average caloric intake = 19,312 / 7 = 2,759 calories

I'm fully aware that some dieters will not want to wait a full week to diet, and therefore I developed a second option of the great metabolism test. Simply get out a pen and paper, write down what you ate and drank yesterday, and count your calories for the day. The next step is to examine the food you ate and ask yourself if this is your typical pattern of eating. If it's a weekend or a holiday, it may involve eating more calories than a normal weekday. That's fine because you can combine a high-calorie day with a lower-calorie day and still get an estimate of your average caloric intake. If it was a high-calorie day, then also write down what you ate and drank in an ordinary day and count your total calories. Divide that total by two to calculate your average caloric intake. An example is listed below:

Monday–Low-calorie day: 1,800 calories

Sunday–High-calorie day: *3,200 calories*

5,000

Average caloric intake = $\dfrac{\textit{Total calories}}{\text{Total days}}$ = 5,000 / 2 = 2,500 calories

This test will discover the amount of calories you need in order to maintain your weight. It will therefore also be used to determine your projected weight loss. If you find that you are eating a lot more calories than you thought you were, that's great news. This means you can consume more calories than you ever imagined and still lose weight. Congratulations! The amount of weight you lose is entirely up to you. You are in control of this program. I'm your coach, trainer, motivator, and teacher. Just use my 22 years of experience to help make the road to thinness a pleasant country drive, not a traffic jam!

I will continue with the example shown above to illustrate that the amount of calories you decrease will in turn determine how much weight you lose.

PROJECTED WEIGHT LOSS ANALYSIS

Average caloric intake	Diet caloric intake	Weekly weight loss	Yearly weight loss
2,700	2,000	1.4	up to 72.8 lbs.
2,700	1,700	2	up to104 lbs.
2,700	1,500	2.4	up to125 lbs.
2,700	1,200	3	up to156 lbs.

As shown by the chart listed above, this client only needed to cut out 700 calories a day in order to lose up to 72 pounds in only one year. That's only 26 percent fewer calories than they were eating before they started this diet!

Now that you have an instant assessment of your caloric intake, you can start your diet today. If you're like the person in the above example, and you start consuming 1,500 net calories a day, you should lose 2 - 4 pounds (if not more) in only 7 days! The magnificent breakthrough in metabolic science is the fact that it's not relative to what you "should" eat in order to lose weight; it's about what you were eating! There's a fine line between obesity and normal weight, and it's those minor changes over a period of time that actually yield permanent weight loss. Now that you are no longer in the dark, let's shed some dietary light upon your individual caloric requirements.

It takes 3,500 calories to equal a pound of weight change; therefore, every time you subtract these calories from your average caloric intake, you will yield a one-pound weight loss. This is based on science and defines the base line for weight loss. (You will also lose more weight depending on your level of activity.) The *least* amount of weight you will lose is based upon this figure. I have had clients lose 13 pounds in one week, and it's obvious that they did not negate 45,500 calories from their normal intake in only 7 days.

FOOD AND BEVERAGE DIARY

The most important thing you can do for yourself during the first week of dieting is to get into that ongoing habit of writing down what you eat and drink on the same day that you consume it. When you keep a daily food diary, you can study your eating habits and troubleshoot your problems very quickly. For instance, if you discover that you often devour a bowl of chips after dinner, you can then begin to capture this snack culprit by beating it at its own game. Begin by mixing in a lower-calorie munchie, and then gradually cut the snack size in half with a smaller bowl. Eventually you'll no longer crave these high-fat snacks because you desire thinness more than you want junk food.

It's so enlightening to write down what you eat. The reason why your food and beverage diary must be completed each day is twofold. First, you need to be aware of your caloric intake before dinner so that know how much you can eat that evening. I've had clients realize, after reviewing their diary, that they already ate over 1,000 calories during breakfast and lunch.

I look forward to adding up my first two meals, which, you'll remember, I go very light on so I can have a delicious dinner or a nightly snack. If you say that you won't go out to eat and all of a sudden you find yourself out on Friday night with a menu in one hand and a beer in the other, don't get upset with yourself. Instead of telling yourself it won't happen, plan for it to happen in advance.

The second reason is that we need to be held accountable for what we eat. You may want to forget about writing down some snacks, cakes, cookies, and ice cream, but the scale will not forget it. Most dieters don't even know how many calories they require per day to maintain their weight. Think of it as a lifelong lesson. As you review your food diary, you will see your eating patterns, as well as which food contributes the most to your total caloric intake. The practice of writing it down also teaches you to eliminate wasted calories. If you see that you ate four cookies at work throughout the day, then you may think twice about doing it again. If each cookie is 100 calories, you just wasted 400 calories without feeling full.

You deserve to be normal weight. Once you review your food trends, you can make logical decisions about how to change your diet so you can lose weight on a weekly basis. Now is the time to be your own diet detective and figure out where you can eliminate calories without subtracting volume. My clients actually eat more volume now than prior to dieting.

INSTRUCTIONS FOR FOOD AND BEVERAGE DIARY

1. Always be specific when writing down what you eat. Include:

   - What you ate, as well as the amount.

   - Where you ate it (optional). Some dieters like to see where they ate, such as at home, with friends, family, or at a restaurant.

2. If you don't know the calories of the food, don't take a wild guess. Look up a similar food in your calorie-counting book to get a rough estimate. If

you do guess, then indicate on your diary that you're not sure by putting a question mark next to the number of calories.

3. Make sure to record all portion sizes very carefully. This can make a difference of thousands of calories by the end of the week. If you don't know the exact size, then estimate to the best of your ability.

4. Include beverages. Remember to write down everything you drink each day. Get yourself into this habit by keeping your recording chart somewhere handy, like on the refrigerator, and writing down what you eat immediately after you eat it. Later in the day, you may forget that you consumed extra food if you didn't write it down. Remember that your scale, however, won't disregard this additional food.

5. The diary will help you understand the reason for your success, as well as how to make changes in your eating habits when you're not losing weight. Here's an example of one diary that conceals the facts, and another that reveals the calories truly:

WRONG:

	Food	Amount	Calories
Meal 3	Spaghetti Meatballs Salad Bread		200 50 50 50 350
Beverages	Soda		100
			Total Calories = 450

RIGHT:

	Food	Amount	Calories

Meal 3	Spaghetti
	Meatballs
	Grated cheese
	Italian bread
	Butter
	Tossed Salad:
	    Lettuce
	    Tomato
	    Cucumber
	    Cheese chunks
	    Croutons
	    Italian Dressing
		2 C.
		2 large
		2 Tbsp.?
		1 slice
		1 Tbsp.
		
		1 C.
		½
		1 C.
		1 oz.?
		¼ C.
		2 Tbsp.?
			320
			800?
			54?
			80
			100
			
			5
			12
			10
			100?
			50
			160?
			<u>1,691</u>

Beverages	Orange Soda	10 oz.	125
Total Calories = 1,816			
The first diary was off by 1,366 calories!			

Get into the good habit of honestly recording your eating and drinking each day. You can use a diary format similar to this sample.

Food and Beverage Diary			
Date:_____			
	Food	Amount	Calories
Meal 1			
Meal 2			
Meal 3			
Meal 4			
Beverages			
Total Calories =			
Date:_____			
	Food	Amount	Calories
Meal 1			
Meal 2			
Meal 3			
Meal 4			
Beverages			
Total Calories =			

DON'T TEMPT ME

If you feel that a certain food sends you over the edge, this means that you are not ready to eat it. When you're in line at the store and ready to check out, staring right at you is your favorite candy bar, and the thought runs through your mind, *I haven't eaten that in a while; why don't I just buy one and treat myself? That little candy bar won't cause me to gain weight.* The next thing you know you're driving home and all that is left is the wrapper. Now you feel pangs of guilt because you let your defenses down. This is the time to stop this behavior and go on. Don't let it get you upset. Instead, learn from it. If all you wanted was something sweet to eat on the way home, then find a low-calorie substitute. You could have chewed a piece of gum, eaten a breath mint, or sucked on some hard candy. Don't let your taste buds determine what you eat and ultimately what you weigh. You need to accept the fact that temptations will occur, and it's how we respond that determines our success. You should train yourself to question the food before you act upon an impulse.

One technique used by my clients to control their snack attacks is the party mix theory, described later in this book, and now I'll tell you about another successful method.

THE SMALL PLATE THEORY

The small plate theory is a method of portion control I have taught my clients to use for 20 years. The concept is based upon the fact that as children we are taught to finish what we start. As a child you were probably told to eat your supper, and that means everything on your plate, so that you may have dessert. Our mind is programmed to start at the beginning and stop when the project is done. If you use this mindset with food, it usually leads to dietary disasters. I've asked plenty of clients if they can just eat one small piece of a candy bar and then put it back away. They all replied that once they start eating it, they must finish the whole thing. That's why I recommend the small plate theory. If you start with fewer calories per portion, then it's a fact that you will consume a smaller amount of food. My family used platters on Sunday to serve their pasta, and I started to notice as a child that the larger the plate, the larger the person, thus the reverse also holds true: the smaller the plate, the smaller the person. This theory works especially well for the dieter that's used to taking more than one portion of food. I use a tiny bowl for my evening pasta meal intentionally, because I know in advance that I will be having four helpings of my meal. This means I have to get up and prepare the dish several times, which takes time, thought, and effort. As a result I eat slower and enjoy my meal. I also look forward to the future portions I have entitled myself to.

The perfect example of the small plate theory is from actual diet clients. One person told me that they couldn't stop eating their ice cream, and when I suggested changing to low-fat ice cream or frozen yogurt, they stated that they would accept no substitutions! I replied that I had a perfect solution. Take a small champagne glass, which only holds 4 ounces, so that you begin with fewer calories. Then use your ice cream as a condiment, not the main entrée. Put your favorite sliced fruit on the bottom of the glass and top it with a small portion of ice cream, then top it with a crumbled fat-free cookie and some low-calorie whipped cream. Make a beautiful low-calorie sundae, and go ahead, have another because they're small, not large! The idea of consuming your food in smaller portions is beneficial to dieting in several ways. The most important of these is determining hunger. It takes your body 10–20 minutes after the food reaches your stomach to satisfy your hunger. It is obvious therefore that the slower you eat, the fuller you feel. If you gobble your meal up in 5 minutes, your body barely even knows you ate, and your brain is still sending out signals that tell your body you are hungry. Another advantage of a small plate is the appreciation of food. How many of you eat food to please your taste buds? Do you choose the food because it provides your body with the necessary nutrients in order to sustain life or because it simply tastes good to you? I'm not asking you to be a perfect dieter; just take the time out to enjoy the food you can have.

WEIGHING IN

Now comes the weigh-in. You step on the scale, and you've lost weight. It's at this point that you are instantly rewarded. You are at a vulnerable point in your life right now, because you want to celebrate your accomplishment. If you need to reward yourself, then do it with something other than food. I'll give you a real-life example of two diet clients. One was a teacher and the other a school secretary. They came to their diet meetings together, which can be good or bad. After several weeks of losing weight, I made a joking remark about clients who rejoice in their accomplishments by eating. They both chuckled, and I knew something was up. They admitted to me that every time they lost weight, they drove right down the street to the local fish fry and ordered a meal.

This isn't the most logical thing to do, but people still do it. If you want to binge or eat more than you know you should, then eat another portion of healthy diet food, not junk food. I've asked dieters why they didn't just overeat a bag of nonfat chips instead of the regular high-fat version, and they reply, "If I did, then I wouldn't consider it being bad."

A common question is, "What if I don't lose weight one week? Is there something wrong?" The answer is, "No, but this does not give you the liberty to give up. Remember the goal here!" There are many reasons that this can occur, some of which are listed below. Carefully read through these and decide which of these pertains to your specific situation.

1. Our body weight changes throughout the day. As we consume food and beverages, our weight shifts according to our intake. Our lowest weight is in the morning after going to the bathroom. This is the weight you should report in your diet journal. Experiment with your own body to understand these fluctuations in weight by weighing yourself before and after drinking water and eating a meal. A change of clothing will also change your weight.

2. Scales only measure total body mass. The scale does not measure what percent of our body is water, fat, and muscle. Therefore the scale cannot show us when we are losing fat and replacing it with muscle, so it registers the same weight. In order for us to know the difference, we must measure ourselves with a tape measure. When we are losing inches, we are losing fat, which is more important than a number on an inaccurate scale.

3. Most bathroom scales are inaccurate for registering small changes of 1 or 2 pounds. Sometimes stepping off and back on will change the weight.

4. The amount of sodium (salt) that we eat each day can drastically influence our weight. The more sodium we consume, the more water our bodies hold. Therefore an increase in sodium intake can cause a gain of water weight. When we reduce the sodium intake and increase the water intake, our weight will also reduce.

5. Women should understand that their weight fluctuates every month during menstruation. Symptoms include abdominal bloating and weight gain. This weight gain is only water and can show up on your scale before, during, and for a short time after your menstrual cycle.

6. Losing weight is different for each person because our bodies respond to reduced caloric intake differently. For instance, a person may lose 5 pounds one week and none the next week. This is an average of 2.5 pounds per week, which is just the right amount of weight reduction for permanent weight loss. The reason the scale shows no weight loss the second week

is because the first week could have been 2 pounds of fat and 3 pounds of water. The next week those 3 pounds of water could simply have been restored while the body also lost 3 pounds in true body fat, and the scale will obviously show no apparent weight change that week. The important point here is that your body truly lost 2.5 pounds of fat each week, which brings you closer to this important goal.

Note: If none of the reasons listed above apply to you, then it is time to take a good look at your food and beverage recording charts. Monitoring yourself carefully is the most important part of your weight-loss program. You should read the checklist and make sure you are following the proper directions for your food and beverage recording chart.

1. Do you write down what you eat shortly after you eat it? If not, how can you remember what you ate last week, let alone the exact portion sizes? Get yourself into the habit now; you'll appreciate it later.

2. Did you accurately record all portion sizes? Increasing the actual amount, or just taking a wild guess, will only make it take longer to achieve your weight-loss goal. Start measuring your portions of higher-calorie food and use measuring cups, spoons, and a diet scale.

3. Are you counting your calories properly? If you eat more than one serving of a food, make sure you multiply the calories per serving by the number of servings you consume. If you have had 800 calories for the day and go out to a party and snack on munchies, don't tell half-truths by writing down only 400 calories in your journal and magically come up with a perfect 1,200 calories for the day.

6. BREAKING THE RULES

You won't see flashing lights in your rearview mirror, nor will you be issued a yellow ticket to appear in court, because the rules I'm talking about breaking are traditional diet laws.

1. THE MOST COMMON DIET DECREE IS THAT YOU SHOULDN'T EAT AT NIGHT.

Some weight loss programs have the nerve to tell the dieter what time to go to bed at night. The specific nighttime food restrictions vary, depending on which diet book you pick up off the shelf, but the message is a stern one, even though the consequences are not quite clear. The concept stems from the assumption that the dieter has already consumed all of her allotted calories for the day, and the additional consumption of calories would put her over her daily limit and in turn hinder her weight loss.

It's disconcerting enough to be told what to eat, but then the author goes one step further and tells you when you can consume their often-meager menu selections. The whole concept of munching to the clock can be counterproductive to weight loss for several reasons. The foremost of these is that your brain thinks it's time to eat, even if you're not hungry. You wake up in the morning and feel pressured to eat breakfast because you've been told that it's the most important meal of the day. I have a sneaky suspicion that a company that sells breakfast cereals started this rumor. The incentive to eat upon rising is based upon social pressure, especially in the United States. The diners and donut shops are hustling and bustling with business from six a.m. on. These establishments are full of consumers who justify their consumption of a high-calorie meal because they need to eat breakfast. Although breakfast is important, that's no reason to declare it supremely essential and then exploit that concept by over-eating the wrong foods.

If you're still under the assumption that your first meal of the day is the most important one, then why are so many Americans fulfilling their dietary requirements by purchasing fast food and eating at "greasy spoon" restaurants? If it were so important to them, then why not at least have a nutritious one? It's plainly and simply diet justification. When a dieter convinces herself and others that she's eating because it's the right thing to do, then it provides her with the justification to proceed with the action.

If you consume the majority of your calories during the day in hopes that you'll refrain from eating anything else the rest of the day, it's important to remember that temptation can foil even the best laid plan. You don't want to put yourself in a situation where you can't have too many calories at a cocktail party or social occasion because you didn't plan your caloric strategy correctly. What I mean is: plan in advance how many calories you'll save for your evening appetizer and meal.

It's a common excuse amongst dieters to blame their nighttime eating episodes as the cause of their weight gain. This is because they are constantly bombarded with diet books that tell them eating at night is taboo and considered a dietary sin! It's time to wipe the slate clean of diet myths. Step up to the plate and recognize when you're being thrown a curve ball. You need not give up your nightlife and go to bed at sunset in order to avoid eating at night. The time you consume your calories doesn't have any significant bearing upon your weight loss. It's the total calories you consume for the entire day that determines the rate at which you lose weight. It's therefore your decision when you want to eat your calories.

Every one of my clients enjoys eating in the evening. This is often a result of cultural habits that their family and friends have practiced for centuries. The recollection of my family sitting around the dinner table conversing and sharing the news of the day comes to mind immediately. That's because it's an important part of socialization and what universally bonds families together. The dinner table is where memories are made. It's time to relax and enjoy the fruits of your labor and appreciate the love and affection that your family brings to the table. If you take pleasure in eating your calories during the evening, then by all means do so. The only stipulation that applies is that you consume fewer calories during the day and plan in advance how many calories you have left to eat at night. In my diary, I consume 1,200 net calories per day and prefer to save the majority of my calories for the evening. I only eat 300 calories before 7 pm. This is done intentionally so that I can bank up my calories and eat the remaining 900 calories at night. This method of eating has resulted in weight loss and eventually allowed me to maintain a weight of less than 100 pounds!

It's not the time of day you eat your calories that determines your weight. Don't let diet misconceptions dictate what time of day you are allowed to eat. This is your diet, and no one knows your schedule or eating patterns better than you do, so go ahead and break the rules. The only penalty you'll have to pay is that you're no longer a victim of mythical diet rules.

brand name clothing was being produced. The average bartender needed the latest cocktail guide in order to stay afloat at their profession. At that point, I realized I was the brunt of the joke, and Anne just chuckled as she exclaimed that sex on the beach was the latest craze in fancy cocktails. Anne described the beverage, and I proceeded to count the calories of the drink so that she would know in the future.

Anne continued to drink alcoholic beverages on a regular basis and lost weight every week. After Anne achieved her 20-pound weight loss goal, she competed in a weight-lifting contest. Anne won her division because of her adherence to the weight-training program that I designed for her. Plenty of my clients drink alcohol and lose weight on a regular basis. The point here is that they were responsible for their intake and counted the calories of the alcohol they consumed. It's up to you to decide how you want to spend your calories. After you've taken the Great Metabolism Test and determined how many net calories you need to consume in order to lose weight, then you can decide how many of those calories you want to consume from alcohol.

Now comes the interesting part of the weight loss equation. All calories are not created equal because of their rate of absorption and digestion in the human body. It's chemically proven that part of the caloric absorption of alcohol is dissipated during the process of intoxication. This means that some of the calories are expended rather swiftly because they are being utilized to initiate the effect of alcohol on the brain commonly referred to as a *buzz*. Still, if you do decide to consume alcohol, make sure that you stay within your caloric limits, and don't use your altered state of mind as an excuse to consume excessive calories.

3. THE THIRD CONVENTIONAL DIETARY COMMAND IS THAT RECIPES ARE TO BE FOLLOWED VERBATIM.

It's as if the instructions are written in blood on stone and the particular items are combined in a mysterious manner that is not to be questioned or modified. The main reason that dieters are hesitant to alter a recipe is because they're afraid that it won't taste the same. I have had clients who will search the world over for a rare spice, and until they find it, they won't prepare the recipe. I felt sorry for these clients and decided to help them overcome their "reciphobia." I coined this term for dieters who are afraid to prepare a recipe unless they follow the directions exactly.

My solution to the dilemma was simple yet unique. I instructed my clients to bring in their favorite recipes that they felt were unsuitable to prepare and eat while dieting. Then I was going to do the unthinkable, which was to take their high-calorie recipe and render it a diet one without ever tasting or preparing it in advance! They say that necessity is the mother of invention, and that's exactly what happens when you long to eat a recipe that you thought was forbidden while dieting. My dieters were thrilled with this new service I offered, so each week they would bring a taboo recipe and anxiously wait for me to give it a caloric makeover. One of the keys to successful dieting is to be able to enjoy the food you love without adding useless high-calorie items that don't contribute to the taste of the recipe.

Now here's how you can transform your traditional recipes into delicious gourmet diet meals. The first step is to write down your family's most common recipes that you prepare on a weekly basis. We tend to be creatures of habit when it comes to cooking, because "you crave what you eat." Once you've put your actual recipe into print, it's time to discern the ingredients and become your own *recipe detective*. This calls for paying close attention to detail, which differentiates a good private eye from a great one! The best way to analyze your recipe is to look for the items that have the highest caloric density. For example, it's important to count the calories of the cooking medium you use to prepare your meal. It's a common mistake of rookie dieters to add up the calories of the meal and disregard the fact that they used a cup of oil to cook the recipe. The most obvious diet offenders are oil, margarine, and butter. That's because fats all contain nine calories per gram versus carbohydrates and proteins, which have only four calories per gram. When you subtract fat from a recipe, it doesn't affect the taste, but it certainly decreases the caloric content of the recipe.

The most logical place to start breaking the cooking rules is with bakery products. They contain the highest caloric density per ounce due to the fats that are added in order to prepare them. The primary dessert that is in dire need of caloric reduction is the all-American cake. I know our brains have been trained to think pie is the classic American dessert, but by actual statistics, the United States consumes much more cake. What was served at every birthday party you ever attended? After reviewing diet journals for twenty years, I would have to say that dieters always seem to underestimate the calories of a piece of cake. This happens for two reasons. The first and foremost is due to the discrepancy in portion size. The average piece of cake is usually double the allotment size that is stated on the label. This translates to double the calories, which most dieters don't account for because they just assume that their serving is one piece of cake.

This book was written to tell you the truth, and you deserve to know the truth about cake, because the knowledge will last you a lifetime. The sooner you are told the reality of the hidden calories you consume, the easier it will be to make lower-calorie choices in order to maintain your weight loss. The actual portion size of a single serving of cake is shown below. Now I know how the term *sliver* was coined!

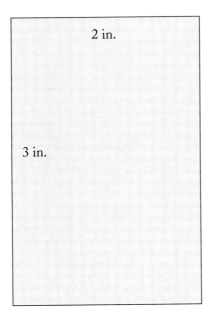

2 in.

3 in.

This is a single serving of cake shown as actual size, which contains approximately 663 calories.

The second common reason for the miscalculation of cake calories is that the dieter glances at the nutrition box and counts only the calories stated on the cake mix. After all, this seems to be the proper way to calculate the calories. What could possibly be wrong with the label? The label isn't wrong per se; it's just the method of marketing that determines how a label is printed. It's a perfect example of "let the buyer beware." The company is fully aware that its product will appear to be lower in calories when they state the calories of the mix only instead of the total calories of the entire recipe. It's up to you to read the fine print and add the additional calories in order to determine the total calories of the cake. Let's inspect an actual cake and frosting mix label and determine the true calories of the recipe as prepared according to the package's instructions. The name of the company is withheld to protect the guilty.

Devil's Food Cake Mix	Calories
Serving Size: 39 g	
Calories per serving: 140	
Servings per container: 13	140 x 13 = **1,820**
Baking Directions:	
1 C. + 2 Tbsp. milk	169
½ C. oil	960
3 eggs	300
Oil or fat to grease pans	<u>240</u>
	1,669
Total Cake Calories =	**1,820 cal**
	<u>+1,669 cal</u>
	3,489 cal
Chocolate Frosting Mix	**Calories**
Serving Size of Mix: 1 Tbsp. (21 g)	
Calories per serving: 80	
Servings Per Container: 14	80 x 14 = 1120
Mixing Directions:	
2 ½ Sticks margarine	2,000
2 Tbsp. milk	<u>19</u>
	2,019
Total Frosting Calories =	1,120 cal
	<u>+2,019 cal</u>
	3,139 cal

Now let's take a look at the label's version versus the genuine finished product.

Presumed Calories		True Calories	
Cake	1,820	Cake	3,489
Frosting	<u>1,120</u>	Frosting	<u>3,139</u>
	2,940 cal		**6,628**

The total calories of this cake with the frosting are 2.25 times the amount that's stated on the labels. Some packages inform the buyer that the calories are for the

"Mix Only," but those words are put on the top of the nutrition facts box instead of being placed in the box. The purchaser therefore has to scrutinize the label with precision in order to obtain an accurate calorie count.

The next distortion of reality in regard to the calories of a piece of cake is the fact that the portion size as stated on the label is not the typical dimensions that are served to you in the real world. A perfect example is to ask yourself how many people actually cut an 8-inch cake into 12 pieces? Now that you are an informed dieter, it's time to make a dietary decision concerning your consumption of cake. You have two choices at this juncture. The first option is to eat a real single serving of cake and dock yourself 600 calories. If you consume the cake at a restaurant, coffee house, or birthday party, you should count the calories as 130 per ounce. It's paramount to dieting success that you should decide that a particular item is worth the calories before you eat it, not after you consume the food. If the piece of cake weighs eight ounces, at 130 an ounce it will be 1,040 calories! Let's say for instance that you are consuming 1,500 calories per day, and you eat a piece of cake that's 1,000 calories. This equates to having only 500 calories left for the rest of the day. When you think of it logically, this dessert isn't really tempting after all.

The second choice you have is the wisest one because it allows you to eat your cake without having to give up a predominant portion of your daily caloric allotment. This is where you'll start breaking the rules in order to lower the calories of the cake. It's interesting to note that according to Webster, the definition of cake is: a baked food made from a mixture of flour, sugar, eggs, and flavoring. There's no mention of oil, which is used in almost every cake recipe in America. So in retrospect what you're really about to learn is to bake a cake according to its definition. The optimum way to give this decadent dessert a caloric makeover is to subtract the items that are calorically dense and aren't required in order to prepare the recipe. The obvious offender in this particular case is the oil. It contributes most of the calories to the recipe and can easily be eliminated without sacrificing any flavor whatsoever. The simplest replacement for oil is water. The major reason oil is added to the recipe is to provide moisture, which is just as easily accomplished by using water instead. This trivial substitution negates 960 calories from the cake and renders it a tad more diet friendly.

The next item that needs to be changed is the frosting. It's mainly compromised of sugar and butter, so the goal here is to find a sweet and smooth replacement to adorn your cake. There are several products that fit these criteria, and the most versatile is low-calorie non-dairy whipped cream. This is a useful item because it fits the bill as being both sugary and provides the proper texture without adding an exorbitant amount of calories to your recipe. The additional benefit to using whipped cream as your cake topping is that it's firm enough to add fruit. It's always a clever dietary decision to put fruit on your cake because raw food provides enzymes and fiber, which are both beneficial to weight loss.

The beauty of knowing how to break the rules of baking is that the recipes you prepare are all new, which allows your palate to develop tastes that are more sophisticated. Now let's look at the revised version of the cake recipe. It's fitting that before the caloric makeover, the cake was called devil's food. After its redemption, this cake could be referred to as dieter's food.

Dieter's Delight Cake	Calories
1 package chocolate cake mix	1,820
1 C. skim milk	80
½ C. water	0
3 eggs	<u>300</u>
Total Cake Calories:	**2,200**
Optional	
Small amt. of spray oil to grease the pan	
Tasteful Toppings	**Calories**
10 Tbsp. low-calorie non-dairy whipped cream	100
2 C. sliced strawberries (or any other desired fresh or froz.en fruit)	<u>60</u>
Total Topping Calories:	**160**
Grand Total Calories:	**2,360**

The original recipe contained 6,628 calories! If each cake is cut into ten pieces, the high-calorie recipe is 663 calories per slice, and the lower-calorie option is only 236. If a person consumes one piece of cake per week, he or she will save 22,204 calories by the end of the year.

4. THE FOURTH EDICT THAT DIETERS FEEL A NEED TO OBEY IS THAT CERTAIN FOODS REQUIRE THE PROPER CONDIMENT IN ORDER TO TASTE GOOD.

This habit is usually cultivated during childhood. As a youngster you are taught that ketchup belongs on your french fries, mustard is for your hot dog, and tartar sauce goes on your fish fry. When you're served a meal at a restaurant, they automatically put the politically correct condiment next to each food item. You need not make an effort to ask for gravy with your mashed potatoes and roast beef, because it's included with the meal. If you were at a psychiatrist's office and they used word association therapy with condiments, you would spontaneously respond to the condiment with a food that it's supposed to be served with. The answer to the word association query is dependent on the country in which you reside. If, for example, you ask a person in England what goes on top of french fries, they would reply vinegar, not ketchup. If you order a pie (pizza pie) in Italy, it may not come to the table with tomato sauce because Americans were the ones who decided tomato sauce belongs on pizza. We adhere to particular food rules because we mistakenly think it must taste better when we eat it that way. It's a travesty that most people don't expand their taste horizons and experiment with new accompaniments for their traditional fare.

Now is a perfect time to take a positive step toward developing innovative ways of adorning your food instead of adding the monotonous toppings you've been using for countless years. If you stop and think about it, what you're really doing is becoming a gourmet diet chef. There are numerous famous chefs with popular cooking shows, yet they have never prepared a low-calorie gourmet recipe. What would these expert cooks prepare if they couldn't use heavy cream, butter, oil, or sugar? If they actually had to pay attention, to how many calories were in their recipes, what would they concoct? It's not difficult to invent a low-calorie dish; mainly these chefs adhere to traditional methods of preparation in order to appeal to the public. This results in a larger audience, which in turn translates to a higher rating for their show. The more popular the program, the higher the cost of advertising becomes and thus more money in the station owner's pocket. Enough about the politics of cooking shows. It's time to become your own gourmet diet chef and break the condiment rules.

First, determine the highest calorie condiment that you use on a consistent basis. The three worst offenders are oil, butter, and margarine. It's essential to remember that it's not only what goes on top of your food that increases your caloric intake; it's also what goes under your food. The oil that you cook with must be added to your calorie count, and once you start doing the math, you'll realize that it's not worth the calories.

There are plenty of non-stick cooking utensils on the market that will eliminate the need for cooking oil. There's a general rule of thumb I teach my dieters in order to determine which condiments they decide to use. *If you can't taste the calories, then don't waste the calories!* The goal here is to be able to invent livable options in order to enjoy your favorite foods and still lose weight.

The reason you need to develop new cooking methods is so that you don't go to extremes for lack of imagination. A perfect example is an actual client of mine who decided she was going to give up all the condiments in order to save calories and facilitate her weight loss. This dieter didn't heed my words of wisdom because she felt that she could pull the old one-upsman on me and go above and beyond the call of dietary duty. This client normally prepared her vegetables in a skillet with oil and then topped them with butter or the latest trendy fat spread on sale at the market that week. I gave her several low-calorie options to adorn her veggies with, but she was vehement about her decision to negate every possible calorie she could and decided to nuke them and eat them plain.

The result was as I had expected. This client became the picture perfect dieter and ate her vegetables because it was the proper thing to do while dieting. It seemed as if she was on the right track, but there was one pitfall she hadn't anticipated. It's a fact that you only continue to eat certain foods when you enjoy the way they taste. Even the most worthy diet endeavor can go astray when it's not properly employed. It's common for dieters to omit condiments altogether, because they lack the knowledge to make an appropriate low-calorie substitution. This leads to diet sabotage because the dieter stops eating low-calorie foods because of their bland and boring method of preparation. *One of the most important aspects of successful dieting is to feel like you're cheating when in reality you're not.* When I tell my diet clients this advice, they look at me as if I've just spoken an oxymoron. The truth of the matter is plain and simple. If you're accustomed to eating in a certain manner and all of a sudden you try to change your whole routine, your defense mechanisms will start to emerge.

The goal is to learn to lower the calories of the foods you love so that you can still eat the recipes and lose weight simultaneously. It's up to you to create unique and palatable substitutions for your dieting pleasure. There's never been a better time to diet, because the food industry is producing new low-calorie food items at a rapid pace. The condiment sections of a natural or gourmet food store provides a multitude of options for a dieter. There are selections from around the world that would turn an ordinary meal into an extraordinary feast. The main criteria you should consider when purchasing the condiment is the total calories of the entire bottle, because portion sizes are usually a lot smaller than the average person consumes.

5. REDUCING THE CALORIES BY DILUTION IS A VIABLE OPTION FOR CONDIMENTS THAT ARE HIGHER IN CALORIES THAN YOU DESIRE.

This is easily accomplished with creamy salad dressings. You can dilute them with skim milk, vinegar, or water depending upon the particular taste of the dressing. If, for example, you cut the salad dressing with an equal ratio of water to dressing, you will decrease the calories by 50 percent!

6. THE OPTIMUM MANNER TO DECREASE THE CALORIES OF A DIET-UNFRIENDLY CONDIMENT IS TO DRAIN THE OIL FROM IT.

This way you can savor the flavor of the food without the added fat and calories. There are numerous gourmet items that fit into this category and are often avoided by dieters because they're packed in oil. The best way to remove the oil is to place the product in an upright position at room temperature so that the oil floats to the top. This method is useful for pesto and nut butters because the remainder of the product stays in the container. If you pour the oil off the peanut butter or nut butters, you can replace the moisture by adding pure water to it and blending it in until you achieve the desired consistency. The second means of removing the oil is to empty the contents into a colander and allow the oil to drip out until it's gone. This process is useful for items such as sun-dried tomatoes, roasted red peppers, artichoke hearts, olives, and marinated vegetables.

After the oil is removed, the best way to calculate the revised calories of your food is to use two pertinent numbers, the calories and fat grams. Let's look at some examples of common foods packed in oil. The first is sun-dried tomatoes, which are extremely high in calories if left in their original state. This caloric makeover allows the dieter to indulge without the bulge.

EXAMPLE 1: SUN-DRIED TOMATO HALVES

Diet Unfriendly	Diet Friendly
(as packaged)	(with oil drained out)
Servings per container: 21	Servings per container: 21
Total calories = 735	Total Calories = 357
Total fat grams = 42	
Total fat calories = $42 \times 9 = 378$	

The next method is used when the product that is packed in oil doesn't contain fat. It's primarily employed for marinated vegetables, which are fat free. If the product itself has fat, then the process of reducing its caloric content is to simply pour the oil off into a measuring cup and subtract the calories based upon the actual amount of oil that's in your measuring cup. The perfect example is natural peanut butter because the oil floats on top of the ground up peanuts, allowing the dieter to drain off the calories from the oil. Let's look at an actual example and calculate the new caloric content of the peanut butter.

EXAMPLE 2: ORGANIC CREAMY PEANUT BUTTER

Diet Unfriendly	Diet Friendly
Serving size: 2 Tbsp.	Serving size: 2 Tbsp.
Servings per container: 14	Servings per container: 14
Calories: 190	**Calories: 155**
Total calories: 2,660	**Total calories: 2,180**

After draining the oil off, the measuring cup indicates 2 ounces have been negated, which adds up to the following in terms of caloric content: 2 oz. x 240 cal./oz. = 480 calories

Now take the total calories of the peanut butter, which equal 2,660 calories, and subtract the calories you drained off, giving you a total of 2,180 calories.

To calculate the revised calories per serving, just divide your total calories by the serving count: 2,180 cal. / 14 servings = 155.7 calories per serving

If you want your peanut butter to maintain its smooth consistency, just add a quarter cup of pure water to it and blend together.

7. YOU SHOULDN'T FOLLOW THE DIRECTIONS, BECAUSE THEY LEAD YOU TO WEIGHT GAIN.

The world's leading food producers don't design their mainstream products to cater to dieters. The cooking instructions are written so that they appeal to the mainstream public. The food industry doesn't care how many calories are added during preparation; they just want you to eat it up and buy some more. The most common ingredients utilized to perfect these recipes are butter, margarine, and oil, all of which are calorically dense and a waste of precious calories for a dieter. The traditional means of cooking is what dieters need to alter in order to render the meal low calorie. This is where we will be breaking the rules in order to consume recipes that would otherwise be "forbidden" while dieting. The predominant enhancers of any meal are the flavor packets. They are a valuable asset to your diet when you prepare them properly. They vary in flavors from gravies and sauces to dips and dressings. A flavor packet can turn an ordinary meal into a gourmet recipe if you disregard the cooking instructions. The best way to explain how to break the rules is to give an example. I've chosen an Alfredo sauce packet because the traditional method of preparation is diet unfriendly.

Alfredo Sauce	Alfredo Sauce	Alfredo Sauce
Prepared according to label directions	Low-calorie preparation	Lowest calorie preparation
Serving size 2 Tbsp.	Serving Size 2 Tbsp.	Serving size 2 Tbsp.
Servings per container 3	Servings per container 3	Servings per container 3
Calories 45 (mix only)	Calories 45 (mix only)	Calories 45 (mix only)
Add the following:	Substitute the following:	Substitute the following:
1 ½ C. milk = 225 calories	1 ½ C. skim milk = 120 cal	1 ½ C. water = 0 cal
1 ½ Tbsp. butter = 150 calories	1 ½ Tbsp. butter sprinkles = 22 cal	1 ½ Tbsp. butter sprinkles = 22 cal
¼ C. grated parmesan = 125 calories		
Added calories 500	Added calories 142	Added calories 22
Actual calories Calories from mix 135 + 500	Actual calories Calories from mix 135 + 142	Actual calories Calories from mix 135 + 22
Total calories 635	Total calories 277	Total calories 157
Calories per serving 211	Revised calories per serving 92	Revised calories per serving 52

The interesting part of the above example is that the calories of the product are listed for the mix only. Therefore a rookie dieter might quickly glance at the sauce packet and count the calories per serving as 45, when in reality the calories per serving are 211, which is 4.6 times higher in calories than the nutritional facts label states! Let the dieter beware, because flavor packets usually list the calories of the mix without adding the additional calories of the items that you use to prepare the finished product!

Salad dressings are the next group of flavor packets that need you to break the preparation rules. They appear innocent until you actually perform the diet math and tally up the total calories of the dressing, as if you adhered to the label directions. The example below depicts various levels of caloric alterations and the resulting reduction of calories that occurs with each substitution. The more willing you are to make modest changes, the more weight you will lose.

Ranch Dressing (prepared according to label directions)	Ranch Dressing (lower calorie version)	Ranch Dressing (even lower calorie version)	Ranch Dressing (lowest calorie version)
Serving size 2 Tbsp.	Serving size 2 Tbsp.	Serving size 2 Tbsp.	Serving size 2 Tbsp.
Servings per container 8	Servings per container 8	Servings per container 8	Servings per container 8
Calories 10 (mix only)	Calories 10 (mix only)	Calories 10 (mix only)	Calories 10 (mix only)
Add the following	**Substitute the following**	**Substitute the following**	**Substitute the following**
½ C. buttermilk 80 cal	½ C.1% fat buttermilk 55 cal	½ C. fat free buttermilk 40 cal	½ C. gourmet vinegar 5 cal *
½ C. mayonnaise 800 cal	½ C.light mayonnaise 320 cal	½ C. fat free mayonnaise 80 cal	½ C. water = 0 cal
Added Calories 880	**Added Calories 375**	**Added Calories 120**	**Added Calories 5**
Actual Calories Calories from mix 80+880	Actual Calories Calories from mix 80 + 375	Actual Calories Calories from mix 80+120	Actual Calories Calories from mix 80 + 5
Total calories 960	**Total calories 455**	**Total calories 200**	**Total calories 85**
Calories per serving = 120	Lower calories per serving = 57	Even lower calories per serving = 25	Lowest calories per serving = 11

* I prefer white champagne vinegar from France, which imparts a slightly sweet flavor, or balsamic vinegar from Italy when you're in the mood for more tang.

The flavor packet story is plain and simple; dieters shouldn't follow the package directions, because they're not intended to be low calorie! It's also imperative to remember that the calories listed on the label are for the dry mix only! There are numerous flavor packets on the market that can enhance any meal when they're prepared using low-calorie culinary tricks. When it comes to lowering calories of any food, *dilution is the solution to your weight loss resolution!*

8. START COOKING WITH WATER INSTEAD OF OIL.

This substitution provides substantial calorie savings without sacrificing taste. If you're accustomed to using oil in your daily cooking routine, it's time for you to get out your measuring cup and see how many calories you're casually pouring into your skillet. It's shocking to most dieters how meager the 2-tablespoon measuring cup actually looks. Now fill the 2-tablespoon measuring device with water and pour it into a pan to compare it to the actual amount of oil you've been using. This amount will not cover the bottom of a 10-inch skillet, which means you've probably been using about 4–6 tablespoons of oil every time you cook with this diet-unfriendly condiment.

If you end up consuming only 2 tablespoons of oil from your recipes, this will add 240 extra calories to your daily intake. If you don't account for this in your food journal, you could end up gaining 25 pounds in only one year! It's paramount to your dieting success that you're aware of the calories that sneak their way into your diet.

It's advisable to purchase or use non-stick cookware when using water to prepare your recipes. The optimum cooking utensils are glass and stainless steel, because they don't contain chemicals that leech into your food. The best way to adapt to this method of cooking is to alter the traditional recipes that use oil in their preparation. If, for instance, you brown some vegetables and meat in oil before adding them to your pasta sauce, it's time to put away the oil and pour on the water. It's actually much simpler to cook with water because it doesn't require constant attention. It's also advantageous because you never have to measure out a particular amount for any recipe; instead, you add it as needed. In the case of the pasta sauce, you just put water on the bottom of the pan and pre-cook your meat and vegetables, then drain off any excess fluid and add the items to your pasta sauce.

The logical reason for cooking with water is *not to waste a calorie if you don't taste a calorie.* If you need to reduce your calories to 1,500 per day in order to lose weight, then why would you want to consume any of them in the form of high-calorie cooking condiments? When you take the time to actually calculate the number of calories that you nonchalantly use when cooking with oil, you'll realize it's a condiment that directly contributes to your weight gain without adding any volume or enjoyment to your daily diet.

9. ORDERING A PIZZA WITHOUT THE GUILT OR THE WEIGHT GAIN.

The main rule of thumb is to forgo the national franchise restaurants because their pizzas could contain considerably more calories than a local pizza parlor. The perfect example of high-calorie pizza is the pan pizza. Everyone who's ever had this type of pie admits that it's impossible to eat without getting your hands greasy because there's so much oil on the bottom of the crust. If you look up the calories in a food value book, it varies according to the year the book was printed, as well as the publisher. It's interesting to note that the more recent calorie-counting books list the calories of the pan pizza higher than their older predecessors. It wouldn't be an issue if they were similar in calories, but the discrepancy is rather eye-catching. The calories varied as much as 50 per slice in two random calorie-counting books. This caloric mystery required further investigation, which I initiated with a phone call to my local Pizza restaurant.

The first person that answered the phone was frustrated and stated that I was asking complicated questions. I asked for the franchise manager and then proceeded to ask him the most important question regarding the calories of pan pizza. The query was: "Is the oil that you use on the bottom of a pan pizza included in the total calorie count of the pizza?" It seems like a simple question for a place that specializes in pan pizza. However, this was not the case. The rationale behind the interview was to determine the actual calories of the pizza so that I could compare their pie to a different local pizza parlor. The more I tried to obtain the answer, the more difficult the endeavor became. I was told several different stories depending upon the restaurant and the specific person who answered the phone.

I decided to go straight to the source and called their corporate headquarters. After hitting several different numbers and listening to numerous recordings, I finally spoke to a real human. The woman was quite bewildered by my request because she just kept telling me to go to their Web site where the calories are posted for each type of pizza. I pointed out that the individual franchise owners use different amounts of cheese and oil for their recipe, so how can you state that the calories are consistent? After explaining myself for the tenth time, she finally got disgruntled and told me to call the restaurant of my choice and ask their cook what the "true" calories of the pizza were. I chuckled and asked her what qualifications this cook would have in order to properly answer my question. The average employee at these fast-food restaurants has probably never counted a calorie in his life, and all of a sudden, I'm supposed to leave my health dangling in the hands of a person who knows little or nothing about the subject matter? I began to wonder how our country let this whole thing get out of hand. It's hard to imagine that our culture let these restaurants serve them day after day, year in and year out, without questioning what they are consuming. These corporations become rich and powerful at the expense of our nation's health.

Next, I decided to speak to the corporate headquarters manager and proceeded to reiterate my request. She explained that there was no one at that office that could decisively answer my questions, and I asked to speak to the person who actually calculated the calories of their pizza. That was absolutely out of the question because they weren't even sure who this so-called person was. I decided to throw a curve ball and asked if the cheese on the pizza was whole milk or part-skim mozzarella. She stated that they don't prepare the pizza at that location, so she didn't know. Why on earth was this the number to call for customer service? I hadn't received any customer service at this point, and I wasn't going to quit asking until I received an answer. She told me that the "real" corporate office doesn't give out their phone number. I asked her how was I supposed to proceed, and she told me that she would put my questions in writing and they would be reviewed in ten business days. I gave her my address and am still waiting for the company to decide whether they are able or legally bound to answer my questions. Many dieters realize they shouldn't patronize restaurants that treat them like a nuisance for asking the caloric content of their food.

The endeavor to discover the actual calories of franchise pizza wasn't worth the aggravation, so I decided to delve into the world of local pizza shops to decide whether their pie was worth the calories. The most favorable type of crust for dieters is comprised of flour, water, yeast and salt, but most restaurants prefer to add a small amount of oil and sugar to the crust to enhance its flavor. Sugar is preferable to oil because it is 48 calories per tablespoon, and oil is 120. You should avoid places that add oil to the dough unless they know it's a very small amount. Otherwise, you don't know how much they put in, and oil has the highest caloric density of any food on earth.

The optimum method of cooking the pie without adding any additional calories is to put the pizza into the oven with an old-fashioned wooden spatula, which negates the need for any pan whatsoever. The general rule of thumb is to take a slice of the pizza and rub your hand along the bottom of it to determine if it's greasy. If the pizza is dry to the touch, then you know there's no additional oil used in the cooking process.

The next step is to order the pizza with the least amount of calories. It's a common dietary mistake to order a white pizza with vegetables and cheese, thinking that it's lower in calories because they omit the sauce and put broccoli or other veggies on top. The white pizza is not lower in calories than a pizza topped with tomato sauce, because they use oil as a sauce instead, which is significantly higher in calories than a red sauce. Therefore, it's best to stay away from white pizza. The most diet-friendly pizza available is a simple cheese pizza.

Another substantial mistake that's commonly made is to purchase chicken wings with your pizza. The travesty of this decision is that it defeats the purpose of trying to economize your caloric intake. The average restaurant-variety chicken wing has approximately 200 calories. As if that wasn't high enough, you add insult to caloric injury by dipping it into the blue cheese that conveniently comes along with every order. The blue cheese dressing has about 100 calories per tablespoon, which equates to 200 calories per ounce! The two together are a diet disaster and should be avoided if you're serious about your weight loss.

Here's a perfect example of why you need not tempt yourself by ordering wings with your pizza. Once I was sitting outside the pizza shop waiting for our pizza, and as I gazed through their window, there was a gentleman eating chicken wings. I couldn't help but notice that with each bite the man dipped the remainder of his chicken into the thick blue cheese dressing. My dieting nature got the best of me, and I started to calculate the actual calories he was consuming. It only took the person five minutes to consume the wings, and during that short time, he ate six wings and four ounces of dressing. That doesn't sound like much for volume, but it certainly adds up quickly in terms of calories. It was 6 wings x 200 calories, equaling 1,200 calories, plus 4 ounces dressing at 200 calories per ounce, totaling 800 calories. Therefore, the total caloric intake for this little side order was 1,200 calories from the wings, plus 800 calories from dressing, which comes to a whopping 2,000 calories! It's only logical to let the wings take flight off your order since they're soaring with calories.

You may want to order your pizza lightly done and unsliced. I know this sounds peculiar, but there's an ulterior motive behind this technique, which allows the dieter to add volume to the pizza at home and to relax and enjoy the meal. Let's say you have the typical family that sets the pizza box on the dining room table and then begins to gobble it up while watching their favorite TV program. Well, it's time to learn the dieter's method of eating a pizza.

The reason for ordering the pizza unsliced is so that you can cut the pizza into more slices than the restaurant does. If they normally cut the pie into eight slices, you can cut it into seventeen slices. The way in which this is accomplished is illustrated below.

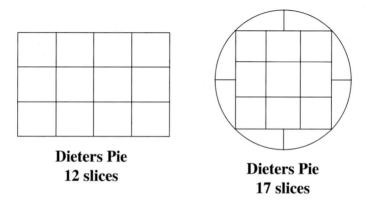

**Dieters Pie
12 slices**

**Dieters Pie
17 slices**

The reason for ordering your pizza with few toppings is that the average pizza parlor doesn't use enough low-calorie condiments. Sometimes they're cooked in oil before putting them on the pizza. It's better to use your own vegetables so that you can accurately calculate your calories. Just add your favorite veggies and warm up individual slices in your oven. This not only limits the tendency to eat the pizza quickly; it also increases both the volume and fiber of your pizza.

Another advantage of customizing your pizza at home is the ability to provide variety. This way everyone in the family can enjoy it because each piece can be customized according to individual dietary requirements and taste preferences. The family members who are dieting can use an array of different vegetables on each piece and turn an ordinary pizza into an extraordinary pizza.

This method of enjoying a pizza allows you to slow down and savor multiple slices. It's depressing to order a pizza then eat one slice and sit there watching the rest of your family munch out. Instead, you've eaten six slices of pizza, and technically, you only had three slices worth of calories. It's gratifying to be able to eat the things that are supposedly forbidden and still lose weight. Once you practice breaking the customary diet rules, you'll wonder why you ever obeyed them in the first place!

10. WHEN YOU'RE IN THE MOOD FOR A SUB, LEARN TO BREAK THE RULES OF ORDERING ONE.

For starters, you'll do well to avoid the national and franchise sub restaurants. The reason for this is twofold. First, these types of places don't cater to dieters. Their goal is to please the mainstream public, and they aren't the least bit concerned about reducing the calories of their submarines. There was one exception where a national sub restaurant ran a marketing campaign that used a couple of testimonies, claiming that eating their subs resulted in weight loss. When you really take the time to research the facts and figures regarding this so-called low-fat sub, it's rather disheartening, or humorous, depending upon whether you believe the stories. After calling several of this company's local sub shops, I was able to obtain the pertinent information. The reality of this sub is that the nutrition facts stated in the commercial are for a six-inch sub with low-fat lunchmeat and without any cheese or dressing. I then asked several employees at various locations how often they sold this type of sub. Their responses were all the same. They indicated that they never sold one of these low-fat subs. The commercial never stated that they were low calorie, which is the number we're concerned with.

The second motive for not ordering from a major sub restaurant is that the ingredients and portions are predetermined and the same for every sub they prepare. It's a simple fact that "special orders" do upset them. The employees are trained to use an exact amount of protein and condiments so that each restaurant is consistent and the customer knows what to expect. Don't expect any exceptions to the rule; special dietary requests are often ignored or scorned.

The optimum place to get a sub is your local sub shop. This is primarily because you can ask them to prepare the sub according to your dietary wishes. It's best to go to a place that has served the community for a number of years, and the owner is available upon request in case you need further assistance. Another incentive for shopping locally is that your purchase really counts, which means that the owner needs your business and will therefore provide excellent service in order to ensure future sales.

Once you've chosen the appropriate sub shop, speak to the person assembling your sub. It's important to let the employee know exactly what you want, so he or she can make the sub according to your specifications. Here are some rules of thumb for ordering subs:

A. Omit tuna salad, chicken salad, and egg salad from your subs. They're prepared using regular mayonnaise, which is 100 calories per tablespoon, and you don't really know how much mayonnaise they've used while preparing them. You're flirting with dietary disaster when you try to convince yourself that mayonnaise-based sub fillings don't contain a lot of mayo. They are simply not built for dieters!

B. Order it without condiments like dressings and mayo. The objective here is to stay in control of the calories in your sandwich. If you allow the employee to put condiments on your sandwich, you won't know the precise amount they've used, so your calorie count will be inaccurate. It's best to avoid guessing your calories, because the average dieter tends to underestimate their intake anyway so that they can eat more. Besides, the typical adornments at sub shops are usually high in fat and can increase the calories of your sub by 50 percent! Instead, you're going to design your own gourmet diet sub. The beauty of this is that you can prepare each section of your sub with different toppings according to your own palate. This creation will provide ample sustenance for two, which means your "sub buddy" can use whatever condiment he or she desires without adding additional calories to your section of the sub. Let's look at the typical condiments used for submarines and the calorie-saving substitutions that can be enjoyed instead.

TRADITIONAL SUB CONDIMENTS

High Calorie Condiment *	Typical Calories for 12" sub	Low Calorie Condiment * (Diet friendly)	Calories	Caloric Savings
Mayonnaise	300	Light Mayonnaise	150	150
		Fat-Free Mayonnaise	30	270
Thousand Island Dressing	270	Low-Fat Thousand Island Dressing	120	150
		Fat-Free Thousand Island Dressing	45	225
Oil and Vinegar Blend	300	Low-Fat Olive Oil Blend	75	225
		Low-Calorie Caesar Salad Dressing	15	285
Italian Dressing	270	Light Italian Dressing	22	248
		Low-Calorie Italian Dressing	15	255
Russian Dressing	240	Light Russian Dressing	90	150
		Reduced-Calorie Russian Dressing	75	165
Blue Cheese Dressing	270	Light Blue Cheese Dressing	75	195
		Fat-Free Blue Cheese Dressing	30	240

* 3-tablespoon Serving

These figures make it obvious that you'll gain an advantage by replacing the traditional high-calorie condiments with your favorite low-calorie dressings.

C. Consider your choice of protein. The best selection calorie-wise is a cheese sub. This negates the high-calorie luncheon meat and allows for the addition of a multitude of raw vegetables. If you have enough calories to spare that particular day and feel an uncontrollable urge to consume meat, then by all means choose a low-calorie option. Then ask the chef to use half the amount that they normally put on a sub. This allows you to savor the meat while still reducing calories.

The whole purpose of this dietary lesson is to enjoy your subs and lose weight at the same time. Our goal is to keep the sub low in calories. Listed below are the high-calorie protein choices that should be eliminated while dieting, as well as the lower-calorie options.

Don't Order		Do Order
High-Calorie Protein Options		**Low-Calorie Protein Options**
BLT (Bacon Lettuce Tomato)	Mixed Italian Sub	Chicken Breast
Bologna	Pizza Sub	Turkey
Chicken Salad	Roast Beef	Cheese
Club Sandwich	Roast Pork	Vegetarian
Corned Beef	Seafood Salad	
Egg Salad	Steak	
Ham	Tuna Salad	
Meatball	Turkey Salad	

It's evident that there are more ineligible subs than there are suitable choices. The point is not to fret over what you can't have but to be thankful for what you can have.

D. Next let's compare our vegetables. These vegetable choices may be found on a conventional sub shop's menu:

Vegetable	Amount	Calories
Lettuce	1 C.	5
Tomatoes	1 C.	20
Cucumbers	1 C.	10
Onion	½ C.	20
Green peppers	1 C.	14
Black olives	1	5
Dill pickle	1	5
Sweet pickle	5 slices	10
Sweet cherry peppers	1	5
Sweet pickle relish	1 Tbsp.	15
Dill pickle relish	1 Tbsp.	10
Red crushed pepper relish	1 Tbsp.	10
Sliced jalapeno peppers	2 Tbsp.	5
Sliced mushrooms	1 C.	14
Yellow mustard	2 Tbsp.	5
Brown mustard	2 Tbsp.	5
Dijon mustard	2 Tbsp.	5
Alfalfa sprouts	1 C.	2

Shredded carrots	½ C.	15
Sauerkraut	½ C.	10
Chopped spinach	1 C.	5
Zucchini slices	½ C.	5
Shredded red cabbage	½ C.	5
Mung bean sprouts	1 C.	10

It's interesting to note that the total calorie count of the entire twenty-four vegetable selections is only 215 calories! It's equally impressive that the combined volume of the veggies is over eleven cups! Now you can significantly increase the size of your sub without adding many calories. The numerous variations and combinations of these vegetables always provide the dieter with plenty of variety.

When ordering your sub, feel free to ask for as many vegetables as possible, and offer to pay for extra ones if you don't have them available at home. Even better, stock your kitchen with your favorite veggies in advance. This way you'll be able to fix yourself a gourmet low-calorie sub anytime.

E. It's always advisable to have low-calorie dressing on hand, and it's available at virtually every store in this country. Do yourself a "caloric favor" and make it a habit to keep several low-calorie dressings in your home, workplace, and any other place where you plan to eat, such as the homes of relatives and friends with whom you often dine. If you're traveling and don't have low-calorie dressing, just order your sub without dressing; then ask for relish, pickles, and mustard on the side so that you can put them on when you assemble your sub.

F. While you're at the sub shop, ask for an extra sub roll. This lets you expand your sandwich options when you get home. Most sub shops are happy to oblige because they buy the rolls fresh from a bakery, and if they aren't used quickly, they're usually thrown away. If you feel apprehensive about ordering an extra sub roll, buy them from a grocery store or bakery before getting your sub. Just be sure to buy low-calorie rolls.

Once you've ordered your sub, it's time to convert it into a diet gourmet sub. You can enjoy your sub cold or warm it in the oven at a low temperature until the cheese melts. (In that case set the lettuce aside until after the sub comes out of the oven.) You can even have your meal prepared both ways, because you ordered an extra sub roll. Take your additional 12-inch roll and divide it into eight pieces. Then take the first sub and move half of everything onto the extra roll. If you do this evenly, each piece remains consistent, and the sandwich becomes a work of art.

If the sub shop didn't have all your favorite veggies, now's the time to add them. This will really turn your creation into a super gourmet delight.

I also recommend cutting the original sub into eight sections like the other one. Then you'll have sixteen pieces instead of one large sub, which tends to be eaten too quickly. The extra pieces also provide dietary satisfaction. How many times have you watched a person order a sub then shuffle off to the nearest seat and gobble it down in a matter of minutes? That's certainly not a memorable eating experience.

Once you've prepared your diet sub, it's time to calculate the calories of your creation. This is best accomplished by itemizing the ingredients and counting their calories individually, in order to achieve an accurate total. The beauty of this method is that once you've analyzed the calories of your sub, you won't need to do it again as long as you order the same item. Here's an example:

ANATOMY OF A DIET CHEESE SUB

Item	Amount	Calories
Sub roll 1	3 oz.	210
Sub roll 2	3 oz.	210
Cheese	4 oz.	280
Lettuce	1 C.	5
Tomatoes	1 C.	20
Cucumbers	1 C.	10
Onion	½ C.	20
Black Olives	5	25
Sweet Cherry Peppers	4	20
Diet Dressing	4 Tbsp.	4 Tbsp. x 11/Tbsp. = 44 cal
		Total calories = 844
		Total pieces = 16 mini subs
		Calories per mini sub = 52.75

8. MENU STRATEGY

The point of changing a recipe is so that you can enjoy it without guilt or putting on weight. I have been serving these recipes at social events for over two decades, and the first response I get is, "Donna, why don't you sell these meals?" Then I reply that my company motto would be *"Her meals are big, and she is not."* When my clients use these recipes, they tell me that the servings are so large that they can't finish them in one meal. So, if you enjoy eating and want gourmet taste without the guilt, get ready to indulge, not bulge! My recipes tend to be Italian, but since I was raised by grandparents from Italy, what do you expect? Italian cuisine is one of the top-selling foods in America. Let's face it, pasta and pizza are crowd pleasers, and we consider them staples in our households.

I'll teach you how to take a high-calorie recipe and turn it into a low-calorie one. We need to take the traditional recipe and discern which calories are worthless, adding no volume or noticeable flavor.

Most diet books fluff up their programs with hundreds of complicated recipes that people never prepare. There is no rule that states you have to prepare a recipe in exactly the manner it was written (see Breaking the Rules). After all, what makes a chef a chef? They don't invent, they just reinvent; they change an ingredient here, a spice there, and voila, you have your very own creation! Many clients have passed up a great recipe because they don't like one of the twenty ingredients in it. You should use the recipe for a baseline and build on it from there. Look at a recipe as a frame, not the whole finished product. What diet book can determine the food you like and then fit it all perfectly into a quick and easy recipe? The trick here is to adjust the formula to your specifications. I will give you a basic format, which you can change to suit your needs. These recipes are designed to be enjoyed by the whole family. You will not have to cook separate meals anymore!

DESIGNER RECIPES

It's time to get into the kitchen and do some gourmet cooking. I would like to point out that it's a relaxing pleasure to cook a meal that I can feel good about and is healthy at the same time. Most of us think good tasting food is the type of cuisine that packs on the pounds and makes us feel guilty in the morning. Not this diet! Your goal is to lose weight, and it will take some time and effort, but so does everything in life that's worth achieving. I can make a diet meal in less time than it takes to put on your makeup. It's time to put things into perspective and think of the benefits you will receive, not to mention the best tasting diet meals you will ever make, and they are so simple to prepare. It's time to reveal the method of cooking these recipes.

The recipe section of this book is built around the four cornerstones of a nutritious diet program. They are pasta, potatoes, rice, and bread products. One of these four items should be the foundation of your main meal, which for most dieters is dinner. Then I tell my diet clients to start the plan in their minds and think of it as four simple items that complete your meal. You have a carbohydrate, a protein, and vegetables. This keeps things in perspective and helps a dieter to design her main entrée according to her level of hunger. When you're more hungry than usual, the trick here is to add volume by using vegetables.

I don't consume my veggies straight up. I sneak them into my meals. If I told you to steam up a bowl of vegetables and eat them plain, you probably wouldn't eat them at all. An excellent example is peppers, mushrooms, and onions. They make a perfect trio. If you happen to like one, two, or even all three of them, they taste delectable when tossed into tomato sauce or a low-fat Alfredo sauce. You need to take the time to write down your favorite vegetables and then take a good look at how you can use them in your recipes. If, for instance, you like broccoli, which is only 20 calories per cup, you can put it on pasta, potatoes, rice, and pizza. This is a bonus because it adds volume with a minimal addition of calories.

After reading over 200 different diet books, which often include numerous recipes, I realized that most dieters don't use that section of the book. One reason is that they often consist of over 15 different items, some of which the reader may not want to eat. How can you really benefit from a diet recipe if you'll never cook it and eat it? *My goal here is to design a recipe system, not a recipe.* You can change the formula according to your likes and dislikes, so everyone can benefit from them.

Let's start with the all important pasta casserole. This recipe is so versatile you can make it once a week for a whole year, and each meal will taste different.

PASTA CASSEROLE

You need to have the proper utensils on hand. So let's take a tour of a diet kitchen. First is the glass-baking dish. It's inexpensive and versatile. It provides a nonstick surface, which negates the need for high-calorie fats. There's no need to fill you up without many calories. This is an example of a low-calorie, good-density food. If you break this down, the potato contains only 15 calories per ounce. The best way to prepare it is steamed, baked, or roasted. The condiments are the key to maintaining a low-caloric recipe. List below are the low-calorie condiments that adorn and complement your potato.

Condiment	Amount	Calories
Light butter	1 Tbsp.	50
Butter Buds	1 Tbsp.	6
Butter sprinkles	1 Tbsp.	15
Low-fat sour cream	2 Tbsp.	40
Fat-free sour cream	2 Tbsp.	30
Fat-free gravy	¼ C.	20
Salsa	2 Tbsp.	10
Grated Parmesan	1 Tbsp.	25
Reduced-fat Mayo	1 Tbsp.	40
Fat-free tomato sauce	2 Tbsp.	15

There are plenty of toppings out there that add a minimal amount of calories to the finished product. So, go ahead and experiment. The recipe should be designed to please you, not the diet author.

RICE

This is an often forgotten grain in the American household, yet it is a staple for other countries around the world. Rice comes in many different varieties and flavors, so experiment and expand your horizons. The exciting part of dieting is to turn your taste buds on to new sensations. Food is meant to provide nourishment, and if prepared properly, it can bestow hours of enjoyment. Most dieters gripe and moan at the thought of cooking rice because it takes 45 minutes to prepare. This can be overcome very simply. Remember that old crock-pot that is collecting dust in your cupboard? Well, now is the time to make good use of it. You can simply get started in the morning before you leave for work, and by dinnertime, it will be ready to turn into a gourmet delight.

Let's turn our sights to the key ingredients that add size to any rice recipe—the vegetables. Listed below are the calories of the top ten vegetables used individually or in delicious combinations.

Vegetable	Amt.	Calories
Broccoli	1 C.	20
Cauliflower	1 C.	15
Water chestnuts	1 C.	50
Bamboo shoots	1 C.	30
Stir-fry sprouts	1 C.	10
Sugar snap peas	1 C.	30
Green beans	1 C.	30
Snow pea pods	1 C.	30
Asparagus	1 C.	30
Mushrooms	1 C.	14

There are obviously more vegetables to choose from, but this is just a quick and easy reference to show you how much volume you can consume if you make wise choices. The rice itself is between 150–200 calories per cup. The best choice is obviously brown rice. If you're not ready to eat as healthy as this, start with white rice and gradually mix half of it with brown, which provides more nutrients and looks rather pleasing to the eye. The key to success in this recipe is to use a condiment without added fat and excessive calories. When it comes to rice, the options are almost endless because the rice will take on the flavor of the sauce or gravy that you put on top of it. Listed below are the ten most commonly used condiments for rice and their calories.

Condiment	Amount	Calories	Amount	Calories
Salsa	1 Tbsp.	5	¼ C.	20
Soy Sauce	1 Tbsp	10	¼ C.	40
Peanut Sauce	1 Tbsp	35	¼ C.	140
Sweet 'n Sour Sauce	1 Tbsp.	25	¼ C.	100
Teriyaki Sauce	1 Tbsp.	20	¼ C.	80
Curry Sauce	1 Tbsp.	30	¼ C.	120
Szechuan Sauce	1 Tbsp.	10	¼ C.	40
Brown gravy Sauce	1 Tbsp.	10	¼ C.	40
Tomato Sauce	1 Tbsp.	20	¼ C.	80
Cheese Sauce	1 Tbsp.	25	¼ C.	100

The next step is to add more volume to the meal by using vegetables. The choice of veggies is based upon your level of hunger and the protein source that will be part of this meal. The flavors should compliment each other and be something that the whole family will enjoy. The goal is to be satisfied enough so that you won't turn to high-calorie junk food when you're finished with the meal. My recipes are so filling that I go to bed full and don't even feel like eating until 1:00 or 2:00 the next day. Now that's volume! The actual preparation of a meal that involves rice is really up to the individual dieter. The rice may have veggies mixed with it or on the side, and the condiment could be the finishing touch to the meal. The protein source will be used as a side dish or tossed into the rice and vegetables for a simple one-pot meal. Listed below are the lowest calorie protein sources that accompany rice rather nicely.

Protein	Amount	Calories
Chicken (white meat w/out skin)	4 oz.	200
Shrimp	4 oz.	120
Scallops	4 oz.	100
Salmon	4 oz.	160
Tuna	4 oz.	120
Baked tofu	4 oz.	120
Beans	4 oz.	70 *
Fat-free cheese or low fat	4 oz.	180
Vegetarian chicken product	4 oz.	120
Vegetarian beef product	4 oz.	120
* = Net calories		

If you're not quite ready to go completely raw as discussed in the chapter Get Raw try steaming your evening meal. Remember that the less time you steam the food, the more nutrients and enzymes will be retained. When I use the term steam, I don't mean using a microwave. This process of cooking deforms the molecular structure of food and in turn destroys the nutrients and enzymes as well! I'm not instructing you how to cook your food, but if you want to obtain the nutritional attributes of steaming food, then the item needs to be steamed, not microwaved.

If you have a steamer, get it out of the cupboard and discover the delicious flavor of steamed vegetables. If you don't have one, then treat yourself to a real steamer. I don't know how I ever lived without this remarkable gadget. The taste of corn on the cob that's steamed will indeed convince you why it's called sweet corn. A steamer is the perfect way to make a delicious one-pot meal. It also generally comes equipped with a rice bowl. The beauty of this appliance is that it's fail safe. The rice doesn't burn, and the vegetables will steam at the same time you're cooking the rice.

There are several cuisines that utilize steamed food. The most obvious are Japanese and Chinese. The mainstay of both these styles of cooking is rice. There is no need to limit yourself to boiled white rice because once you've tasted steamed rice; you'll be pleasantly surprised. If you're not quite ready to delve into brown rice, then try mixing it in a 50/50 ratio in order to develop a taste for it. There are numerous types of rice on the market, and each one has its own unique flavor. Listed below are several suggestions of rice varieties:

Arborio	Jasmine	Wild Rice
Brown	Sushi	Rice blends
Basmati	Wehani	

QUICK SALAD IDEAS

It's always a pleasure to prepare and serve a delectable pasta or potato salad, which in our home transforms the kitchen into a salad bar. A salad is of course a dieter's best friend when prepared properly. The beauty of serving these types of salads is that you can vary the vegetables that accompany the salad according to the season. The dieter can choose several varieties of condiments that are suited to the individual tastes of his or her family and guests that are coming to consume the gourmet salad.

The first thing you're going to do is break the rules of preparation. You'll do this even more in the enlightening Breaking the Rules chapter. The primary reason for improving the preparatory rules is to transform an ordinary high-calorie salad into a diet-friendly feast. The main problem with a typical pasta or potato salad is the condiment, which in traditional recipes is regular mayonnaise. The typical prepared salad contains far too many hidden calories for a dieter to consume.

There are numerous advantages to making the salad yourself. The first of them is that there won't be any mystery calories that show up in the form of weight gain the next day when you weigh yourself. The next benefit to a home-made salad is that you'll be able to eat at least twice the volume that you were previously consuming. Another added bonus is that you'll be giving your taste buds a treat because each serving can taste different. In regard to nutritional value, you'll be able to eat your daily allotment of vegetables in one meal. This variety of veggies provides your body with thousands of micronutrients. When you partake of raw vegetables, it stimulates digestion because the raw food contains enzymes. This in turn boosts your metabolism because you digest your food more efficiently. Who would venture to think that there are so many bonuses to such a tasty meal?

The usual manner in which a diet book presents a recipe is by listing the ingredients and then the instructions. This presents several pitfalls for the dieter. The first of these is the mere fact that the recipe will only be prepared by those who prefer the foods used in their concoction. The second limitation presented by a pre-fabbed recipe is the strict adherence to exact formula without offering substitutions. What's a dieter to do if they don't like half the ingredients used in the recipe? That's precisely why most diet recipes never make it to the table. The ideal recipe is a master recipe that provides you with a great foundation on which you can build the salad according to your personal food preferences. The third problem with these types of rigid recipes is that they aren't what I call "family friendly." What I mean is that they often include strange spices and unfamiliar vegetables that you know your family won't eat. The whole point of preparing a low-calorie recipe is so that you and your family can expand your food horizons and lose weight at the same time.

The initial step to preparing a successful salad is to decide whether you're in the mood for pasta or potato salad. The decision may be based upon your level of hunger. When you perform the diet math, it boils down to 250 calories per uncooked pound of potatoes or 60 calories per dry ounce of pasta. They're both a caloric bargain and rank high on the satisfaction chart.

The manner in which you serve these salads will both be the same. The vegetables will be sliced, diced, or chopped and served in individual bowls like a restaurant salad bar. This enables the dieting family members to embellish a salad with the lower-calorie vegetables and allows the entire family to enjoy the meal together without putting any stress on the dieter.

Now it's time to get into the kitchen and prepare a gourmet salad. I'll start with the pasta salad because it's probably the more popular of the two, or perhaps it's because I'm Italian and pasta is a way of life. The shape is left up to your imagination, and the opportunity for variety is what can make the recipe unique every time you concoct it. The choice of pasta should be one that appeals to the family so that you won't have to cook two different pastas. The commonly delectable choice is often a tri-colored fusilli.

The next step on your pasta salad journey is to determine which vegetables will adorn your salad. The decision once again should be to include at least 3–4 different vegetables so that everyone's favorite can be included on the menu. The vegetables can then be cut according to your preference and placed in individual bowls. While you're slicing and dicing the veggies, the pasta should be cooking. It's advantageous to prepare the pasta al dente so that it remains firm when you put on the dressing. The pasta should be rinsed with cold water and then put into a serving bowl.

The next step that you take is what differentiates a high-calorie salad from a low-calorie one. The traditional condiment for pasta salad is regular mayonnaise, which contains 100 calories per tablespoon. The amount of mayonnaise that can be haphazardly put on your innocent fat-free pasta is the diet-disaster culprit of the mainstream pasta salad. In order to avoid this caloric pitfall, all you need to do is alter the condiment to low-calorie mayo, mixed with low-calorie salad dressing, and only use enough to deter the pasta from sticking together.

At this juncture, you may decide upon the type of dressing you want to put on your pasta salad. You need not limit yourself to one condiment, because variety only enhances the flavor of your recipe. There are numerous low-calorie mayonnaise choices available, and they pair perfectly with low-calorie Italian dressing or any low-calorie dressing of your choice. If you're preparing 8 ounces of pasta, you can use as little as 2 tablespoons of each condiment prior to serving your salad. Then toss the pasta with your desired dressing, put in a covered bowl, and chill it until you're ready to serve.

The great thing about the "salad bar" style of serving is that the dieting members of the family can use more of the low-calorie items on top of their pasta and still enjoy ample volume as well as variety. The trick here is to really appreciate your condiments instead of having your pasta drowning in high-calorie oil or mayo.

The anatomy of a diet pasta salad is basically to start with your pasta on the bottom of the dish and then assemble your desired vegetables on top. The condiments then adorn the finished product. This way you're able to appreciate the taste of it and control the portion, which in turn enables you to monitor your caloric intake.

The second type of salad is the potato salad, which is cooked in the same manner as the pasta salad. You should cook the potatoes to their desired tenderness and then toss them into a colander and rinse them with cold water. Then put on a small mixture of low-calorie mayo and low-calorie salad dressing. The only difference is that you'll be using potatoes instead of pasta for the foundation of your salad. Listed below are the low-calorie condiments and vegetables that compliment a pasta or potato salad.

GOURMET SALAD CONDIMENTS

Condiments	Amount	Calories
Light Mayo	1 Tbsp.	50
Fat-Free Mayo	1 Tbsp.	15
Fat-Free Blue Cheese Dressing	1 Tbsp.	50
Fat-Free Caesar Dressing	1 Tbsp.	25
Low-Calorie French Dressing	1 Tbsp.	30
Fat-Free Honey Dijon Dressing	1 Tbsp.	35
Light Italian Dressing	1 Tbsp.	15
Light Ranch Dressing	1 Tbsp.	35
Fat-Free Thousand Island	1 Tbsp.	30

Vegetables	Amount	Net Calories
Artichoke hearts in H2O	½ C.	25
Broccoli, raw (florets)	½ C.	10
Cabbage, raw (shredded)	½ C.	2
Carrots, raw (shredded)	½ C.	15
Cauliflower, raw	½ C.	7
Chick peas	¼ C.	30
Cucumber slices, raw	½ C.	5
Bean sprouts	½ C.	2
Mushrooms, sliced, raw	½ C.	7
Onions, chopped, raw	½ C.	20
Peppers, yellow, green, red, julienne, sliced, raw	½ C.	7
Radish, diced, raw	½ C.	2
Shallots, raw, chopped	1 Tbsp.	2
Soybeans	¼ C.	30
Summer squash, raw, thinly sliced	½ C.	5
Tomatoes, sliced, raw	½ C.	10

GOURMET SALAD TOPPINGS

Ingredients	Amount	Calories
Artichoke hearts (in H2O)	½ C.	25
Sun-dried tomatoes (with oil drained)	5 pieces	25
Black olives	5	25

Green olives	5	25
Bread n' Butter pickle slices	10	10
Cornichons	10	5
Capers	2 Tbsp.	10
Roasted red peppers	½ C.	7
Roasted yellow peppers	½ C.	7
Kalamata olives	5	15
Feta cheese	1 oz.	70
Shredded low fat cheddar cheese	1 oz.	70
Marinated mushrooms	½ C.	15
Dill pickles	1	10
Shredded haloumi cheese	1 oz.	80
Jalapenos sliced	2 Tbsp.	5

When you diet one of the most important factors that contribute to the success of your weight loss is variety. It's time to change the way you envision certain types of recipes, as well as the particular time of year that you are supposed to enjoy a salad. When you think of pasta and potato salad, you automatically associate these salads with summertime. Let me give you a perfect example from my own life. The memories I have of these two salads are ingrained in my mind. I automatically think of Memorial Day because this is the first celebration of summer. I remember peeling potatoes and chopping eggs and onions to prepare the token summer salads. The manner in which our family prepared these recipes would remain the same year after year, which eventually led to taste bud burnout. What I mean is that you're so used to eating the same concoction that you just consume it out of habit. You know that it will be served, and you eat what you're expected to. The salads had to be made with a certain brand of mayonnaise because it was supposed to be the better tasting choice. The whole point here is, how are you supposed to know what tastes more palatable if you don't vary the recipe and give yourself the option to experience new recipes? The ideal plan of action is to "break the rules" when preparing your salads, and start enjoying gourmet condiments that turn a boring side dish into a scrumptious gourmet meal.

DESIGNER DIET

The latest trend in the fashion industry is to purchase designer clothes, but this isn't an exposé on your latest wardrobe choices. This instead is a lesson on the basics of designing your own diet. It's crucial to your weight loss success that you alter your diet according to your individual food preferences.

You need to develop a diet that you can stay on and not feel deprived. The key to successful weight loss is satisfaction. If you're satisfied both physically and mentally, then you can stay on the program. The problem with going on someone else's diet is that it isn't yours. So it's time to put your diet past aside and design your own diet.

The most exciting part about this diet is designing it. If you could eat what you wanted and be full, you would stay on that diet. Imagine eating pizza, pasta Alfredo, and lasagna and losing weight at the same time? It's time to take a new approach to dieting. Don't eat anything unless you really want to and it's worth the calories. I will teach you how to eat the food you love and lose weight at the same time. It's usually the method of preparation that adds excessive calories to the recipes you enjoy. In some cases, you only have to subtract one tasteless condiment from a recipe to render it diet cuisine.

What really matters is how many calories you're eating to maintain your present body weight. For example, if you're consuming 3,000 net calories daily, then lowering the daily intake to 2,000 net calories will still result in a 2-pound weight loss in only one week. I will show by example that small dietary changes over the course of time will result in significant weight loss.

You need to take the time to jot down your most common breakfasts, lunches, and dinners (including beverages) with calories. When you write down your favorite meals, make sure they're what you normally enjoy when you aren't dieting. Next, add the calories of these breakfasts, lunches, and dinners. If you reduce the calories of your breakfast by 100 calories each day, then you'll consume 700 fewer calories every week. Now do this for one year, and you'll lose up to 10 pounds by the end of that year. That doesn't sound like much, but let's take a closer look at the situation.

If you reduce your lunch by 100 calories as well, and then subtract only 200 calories from your dinner, this will save 146,000 calories annually. Now if you subtract 200 calories from any beverage, which could be only 13 ounces of juice, you could lose more than 60 pounds by the end of the year!

Let's review our strategy:

Meal	Daily Net Calorie reduction	Yearly
Breakfast	-100	36,500
Lunch	-100	36,500
Dinner	-200	73,000

Beverages	-200	73,000
Total yearly weight loss up to 62.44 lbs.		**219,000**

BREAKFAST

Your first exercise is to write down your five favorite breakfasts and add up their total calories. Listed below are five examples from actual diet clients.

Breakfast #1	Calories	Breakfast #1 - Diet Version	Calories
1 grocery store muffin	600	English muffin (whole grain)	120
1 C. juice	150	2 tsp. Jelly or preserves	66
1 container regular yogurt	250	2 pats butter	50
	1,000	1 piece of fruit	50
		1 container nonfat yogurt	70
			356

The problem with grocery store and restaurant muffins is the calories. They are much larger than Grandma's version of a blueberry muffin made in a muffin tin. The modern day muffin is really more like a cake batter poured into a muffin-shaped pan and made to look healthy. The flavors tend to give it away. Does a chocolate chip raspberry muffin really sound like diet food to you? You can change from a store-bought muffin to a low-fat or fat-free packaged version and save half the calories. The other option is an English muffin, which contains only 120 calories. Let's take a look at the modified version of this breakfast.

This version saves you 644 calories. If you eat this breakfast once a week, you'll have saved 644 calories times 52 weeks, which equals 33,488 calories, with this one simple substitution!

Breakfast #2	Calories	Breakfast #2 - Diet Version	Calories
1 bagel with ham and cheese at fast-food restaurant	600	1 small bagel	150
1 coffee with cream and sugar	150	2 slices low calorie ham	55
	750	1 medium egg cooked in non-stick pan with	70
		1 slice low fat cheese	25
		1 C. coffee with stevia and 2 Tbsp. light cream	10
			310

The bagel breakfast sandwich above is just one example of making a healthy substitution. When you look up typical fast food or restaurant bagels with breakfast fillings, they range from 500–700 calories if they contain a meat and egg interior. The best substitution is to make your own version. A grocery store bagel is about 150–200 calories and saves you a tremendous amount of calories from fat. There's no need to clog your arteries so early in the day. You can purchase low-fat vegetarian ham slices or turkey sausage to put on your bagel and cook an egg in a nonstick skillet while getting ready for work. If you need to save cooking time, just substitute a slice of low-fat cheese for the egg and save yourself about 250 mg of cholesterol.

If you change to the new version of Breakfast #2 and do this once a week for a year, you'll save 440 calories each week, with only one simple substitution.

Breakfast #3	Calories	Breakfast #3 - Diet Version	Calories
4 small links sausage	354	2 small links low-fat turkey or soy sausage x 60	120
2 slices toast	180	2 slices diet toast	80
2 eggs	268	3 tsp. jelly	60
2 pats butter	66	2 eggs cooked with spray oil in non-stick pan	140
Orange juice	137	1 piece fruit	50
	1,005		**450**

The updated Breakfast # 3 saves you 555 calories every time you eat it. Do this once a week, and you'll save 555 calories over 52 weeks, which equals 28,860 calories per year,

Breakfast #4	Calories	Breakfast #4 - Diet Version	Calories
1 Restaurant style donut	350	4 fat-free cookies x 25	100
1 C. coffee with cream & sugar	150	1 C. coffee with stevia and light creamer	40
	500		**140**

A donut for breakfast is not the optimum way to start the day, but fat-free cookies are a fair compromise. The goal is to make lower calorie choices that yield more volume. This option also keeps you away from the donut shop on the way to work. Many innocent dieters have told me that they just stopped in for a quick cup of coffee, and before they knew it, they left with a donut in their hand. Don't allow yourself temptation. This way you won't have to make a quick decision while under pressure at the drive-thru window.

Breakfast #4 saves you 360 calories each meal. If you use this modified version even one time per week, you'll save 18,720 calories annually.

Breakfast #5	Calories	Breakfast #5 - Diet Version	Calories
Breakfast croissant at Dunkin Donuts	560	1 toaster-type low fat waffle	70
Hot chocolate – medium	330	1 tsp. jelly, preserves, or maple syrup	15
	890	1 pat butter	30
		1 C. fat free hot chocolate	25
			140

I suggest a whole grain waffle instead of a croissant because it's convenient to put into your toaster in the morning. The toppings provide a small amount of fat combined with sweetness in order to mimic a bakery-type item. You save 750 calories every time you eat the new version of Breakfast # 5.

Each dieter has his own unique likes and dislikes. The above examples merely show that small dietary changes will become permanent weight loss. Let's review how many calories and pounds you can lose by the end of the year with only those five meal changes.

	Total calories saved eaten once a week
Breakfast #1	33,488
Breakfast #2	22,880
Breakfast #3	28,860
Breakfast #4	18,720
Breakfast #5	39,000
	Total = 142,948
Total weight loss up to 40 pounds	

Small changes equal permanent weight loss! You will lose up to 40 pounds in one year with only five small breakfast substitutions!

LUNCH

Now onto lunch to see how much more weight we can lose without subtracting any volume or flavor! Here are ten common lunch choices that show you by example how to incorporate the dietary changes into your lifestyle with little or no effort.

Let's take a look at the revised versions of these typical fast-food lunches.

Lunch #1 (McDonalds)	Calories	Lunch #1 – Diet version	Calories
Big Mac	570	2 slices diet bread or reduced calorie	85
French fries (large)	540	hamburger roll	
Soda (small)	150	2 oz. 85% lean hamburger	90
	1,260	3 tsp. diet ranch dressing	20
		2 tsp. ketchup	10
		½ C. lettuce	2
		2 slices tomato	2
		2 slices pickles	1
		3 oz. baked fries	150
		1 diet soda	0
			360

This saves you 900 calories each time you eat the new lunch.

Lunch #2 (Pizza Hut)	Calories	Lunch #2 – Diet version	Calories
Personal Pan Pizza,	813	Diet frozen pizza or pizza pocket	350
cheese Soda (small)	150		
	963	1 salad: lettuce, tomato, cucumber,	50
		green peppers, carrots	
		2 Tbsp. low calorie salad dressing	20
		1 Diet soda	0
			420

The updated lunch saves you 543 calories.

Lunch #3 (Boston Chicken)	Calories	Lunch #3 – Diet version	Calories
Chicken sandwich with	680	2 slices diet bread or low calorie	85
cheese & sauce		hamburger roll	
Coleslaw	300	3 oz. grilled chicken breast	150
Brownie	450	1 slice low-fat cheese	50
Soda (small)	150	2 Tbsp. diet dressing	40
	1,580	(Teriyaki, Honey Dijon, Italian,	
		or French)	
		Salad: 1/2 C. lettuce	2
		2 slices tomato	2
		2 slices raw onion	2

		Cole Slaw: ½ C. cabbage	5
		Grated. 1 Tbsp. low calorie mayo, a sprinkle of vinegar, and 1 tsp. sweetener	60
		1 Fat free, low cal. choc. cookie	40
		1 Diet soda	0
			436

This substitution saves you 1,144 calories every meal.

Lunch #4 (Burger King)	Calories	Lunch #4 – Diet version	Calories
Whopper with cheese	1,010	1 Kaiser roll	150
French fries (medium) Vanilla shake (medium)	400 430	2 oz. lean beef or vegetarian burger	90
	1,840	1 slice low-calorie cheese	30
		2 slices onion	2
		2 slices tomato	2
		2 Tbsp. light Mayonnaise	50
		3 oz. low fat french fries	110
		1 vanilla cream diet soda or flavored seltzer	0
			434

This shaves off 1,406 calories per meal.

Lunch #5 (Taco Bell)	Calories	Lunch #5 – Diet version	Calories
Taco salad with salsa	850	1 small fat free soft tortilla shell	80
Soda (small)	150	1 C. lettuce, chopped or shredded	5
Side order of nachos	760	¼ C. salsa	20
	1,760	¼ C. chopped onions	10
		¼ C. chopped tomato	5
		3 oz. lean ground beef	150
		2 Tbsp. low calorie sour cream	30
		1 oz. shredded low fat cheddar or Monterey Jack cheese	70
		1 oz. fat free nacho tortilla chips	110
		1 diet soda or seltzer	0
			480

This liberates 1,280 calories, and if consumed only once a week, you will save 66,560 calories annually.

Lunch #6 (Wendy's)	Calories	Lunch #6 – Diet version	Calories
Baked potato with cheese	570	1 medium baked potato	90
Breaded chicken sandwich	440	1 pat reduced fat butter	25
Soda (small)	150	1 slice reduced-calorie cheese (such as American, cheddar, or Monterey Jack; if grated use 1 oz.)	50
	1,160	1 low calorie hamburger roll or 2 slices diet bread of your preference	80
		3oz. chicken breast patty	150
		2 Tbsp. low-calorie Mayonnaise or low-calorie Ranch dressing	50
		1 C. lettuce leaves	5
		2 slices tomato	2
		1 Diet soda, no-calorie spritzer, or water	0
			452

This eliminates 708 calories from your caloric intake.

Lunch #7 (Subway)	Calories	Lunch #7 – Diet version	Calories
6" Classic Italian Super sub (without salad dressing and cheese)	668	1 Diet hotdog roll or 2 slices whole wheat bread	100
3 oz. oil and vinegar	300	1 slice low-calorie ham or vegetarian ham	80
1 slice cheese	80	2 slices low-fat salami	120
1 Choc. Chunk Cookie	215	or vegetarian salami	
1 Berry Luscious smoothie	154	8 small pieces sliced pepperoni	80
	1417	2 Tbsp. Diet Italian dressing	50
		1 C. lettuce	5
		4 tomato slices	10
		1 slice low-calorie cheese	50
		1 Raspberry or berry flavored no-cal spritzer	0

		1 fat free, low calorie chocolate cookie	40
			535

This lean Italian sub saves you 882 calories every time you feast upon it.

Lunch #8 (Olive Garden)	Calories	Lunch #8 – Diet version	Calories
Capellini Primavera with chicken	510	1 C. cooked Cappellini	150
2 Bread sticks	280	1 C. mixed vegetables (cooked in water, steamed, or non-stick skillet in a small amount of spray oil)	50
Soda (small)	150	3 oz. chicken breast	150
	940	¼ C. White Gravy Mix or mushroom gravy prepared with water, or a low calorie ranch dressing)	40
		1 low-calorie breadstick	40
		1 Diet soda	0
			430

The revised version of this meal saves you 510 calories.

Lunch #9 (Kentucky Fried Chicken)	Calories	Lunch #9 – Diet version	Calories
1 Extra crispy chicken breast	470	1 Broiled or baked chicken breast	120
1 order potato wedges	280	3 oz. Baked steak fries	150
1 lemon cream parfait	410	1 serving fat free lemon ice	40
1 soda (small)	150	1 Diet soda	0
	1310		**310**

This low-calorie version will conserve 1,000 calories.

Lunch #10 (Arby's)	Calories	Lunch #10 – Diet version	Calories
Big Montana Roast Beef	720	1 Diet hamburger roll	
Large curly fries	600	or 2 slices diet bread	85
1 Garden Salad	280	2 slices low calorie or vegetarian style roast beef	80

	1600	1 slice low-calorie cheese	40
		2 Tbsp. barbeque sauce	30
		2 slices onion	5
		3 oz. baked steak fries	150
		1 C. lettuce	5
		1 C. cucumbers	10
		½ C. tomatoes	10
		2 Tbsp. low calorie salad dressing (such as Italian or Honey Dijon)	25
			440

These dietary changes will save you 1,160 calories every time you consume the meal. *Do this once a week and lose up to 17.2 pounds in only one year.* As you've noticed by now, the ten lunch selections are all from fast-food restaurants. They are examples of high caloric density meals that are also high in fat and cholesterol.

Now let's review our calorie-saving substitutions and get a tally of the total pounds that can be lost by changing lunches only once each week.

Lunch #1	13.4 pounds
Lunch #2	8 pounds
Lunch #3	17 pounds
Lunch #4	21 pounds
Lunch #5	19 pounds
Lunch #6	10.5 pounds
Lunch #7	13.1 pounds
Lunch #8	7.5 pounds
Lunch #9	15 pounds
Lunch #10	17.2 pounds
	142 pounds of potential weight loss

The diet version lunches were provided as an example of how simple it is to subtract well over 500 calories from a typical fast-food lunch. You will feel full and satisfied until dinner. If you were eating the typical fast-food lunch, then the diet version lunches are a perfect way to lose up to 100 pounds with some simple meal substitutions!

THE PARTY MIX THEORY

I'm not asking you to be a perfect dieter; just take the time out to enjoy the food you can have. Another technique used by my clients to control their snack attacks is the Party Mix. Instead of going cold turkey and trying to switch from potato chips to rice cakes, change your snack habits little by little. Even the longest journey starts with the first step and then continues with each and every step, eventually getting you to the finish line—or in this case to your goal weight. The Party Mix Theory is exciting, because the combinations can vary on a daily basis. The idea is to take the higher-calorie snack and cut it with a lower-calorie item, or even two to three other low-calorie munchies. The choice is up to your taste buds. What I appreciate about the Party Mix is the anticipation of eating a couple of my so-called forbidden snack items, which I anxiously look forward to. The concept is mathematically sound and results in weight loss, as well as establishing new dietary habits. I will show you by example the calorie savings of the Party Mix.

Note: Your family, friends, or children can enjoy these snacks together. The non- dieters eat the higher-calorie snacks, and you eat the lower-calories snacks with an occasional nibble of the "taboo" snacks.

Original Snack #1	Calories	Party Mix Snack #1	Calories
8 oz. potato chips	1,200	3 oz. potato chips	450
		3 oz. potato or soy crisps	270
			720
Original Snack #2		Party Mix Snack #2	
8 oz. mixed nuts	1,360	1 oz. dry roasted mixed nuts	140
		3 oz. pretzel nuggets	300
			440
Original Snack #3		Party Mix Snack #3	
8 oz. tortilla style chips	1,200	3 oz. nonfat tortilla chips	300
		1 oz. pretzels	100
		1 oz. flavored, reduced-fat cheese crackers	100
			500
Original snack #4		Party Mix Snack #4	
8 oz. corn chips	1,200	3 oz. baked corn chips	300
		3 oz. Cheddar Soy Crisps	300
			600

Original Snack #5		Party Mix Snack #5	
8 oz. Cheese twists or curls	1,200	3 oz. Nacho Soy Crisps	300
		2 oz. pretzel twists	200
			500
Original Snack #6		**Party Mix Snack #6**	
3 c. cheddar flavored popcorn	380	3 C. reduced-fat microwave popcorn	90
		1 oz. pretzels	100
			190
Original Snack #7		**Party Mix Snack #7**	
8 oz. BBQ pork rinds	1,500	3 oz. BBQ potato crisps or soy crisps	270
		1 oz. sesame sticks	150
			420
Original Snack #8		**Party Mix Snack #8**	
8 oz. Bagel chips	1,120	3 oz. fat-free bagel chips	300
		2 oz. Melba rounds (flavored if desired)	200
			500
Original Snack #9		**Party Mix Snack #9**	
8 oz. Cheese crackers	1,200	4 oz. low-fat mini cheese crackers	440
		2 oz. pretzels or low-fat veggie or wheat crackers	200
			640
Original Snack #10		**Party Mix Snack #10**	
8 oz. potato sticks	1,200	3 oz. nonfat potato sticks	300
		3 oz. pretzel sticks	300
			600

Now let's review the calories that we save with our revised party mixes.

			Calories Saved
Snack #1	vs.	**Party Mix #1**	480
Snack #2	vs.	**Party Mix #2**	920
Snack #3	vs.	**Party Mix #3**	700
Snack #4	vs.	**Party Mix #4**	600

Snack #5	vs.	Party Mix #5	700
Snack #6	vs.	Party Mix #6	190
Snack #7	vs.	Party Mix #7	1,080
Snack #8	vs.	Party Mix #8	620
Snack #9	vs.	Party Mix #9	560
Snack #10	vs.	Party Mix #10 =	600
			6,450 calories saved

If you snack only 20 times in one month, you'll save 12,900 calories. Over a year, that's 154,800 fewer calories, which will yield a weight loss up to 44 pounds just by decreasing your snack calories, not the volume of your snack.

I have concentrated on the salty, crunchy type foods for this section. The next snack substitutions are for those who prefer sweeter treats.

TEN SWEET SNACK SELECTIONS

Snack #1	Calories	Diet Snack #1	Calories
1 C. regular ice cream	600	Slim sundae:	
		½ C. nonfat frozen yogurt or	90
		Low-calorie ice cream	25
		½ C. fruit	25
		1 fat-free cookie crumbled on top	140

To prepare your slim sundae, take a 4-ounce champagne glass and put your favorite sliced fruit on the bottom. Then dollop the low-calorie ice cream on top, and for the finishing touch, crumble your low-calorie cookie on top, or set it on top whole if you prefer. This recipe is large enough to split into 2 servings. Go ahead and treat yourself!

Snack #2	Calories	Diet Snack #2	Calories
1 candy bar	450	1 chocolate-flavored energy bar	200
Snack #3		**Diet Snack #3**	
1 piece pie	500	Dieters' dream pie:	
		1 low-fat graham cracker	45
		½ C. fat-free pudding	75

		2 Tbsp. fat-free whipped cream	15
			135

This pie requires no baking and of course no guilt. You can warm up the graham cracker if you choose to or have the whole dessert cold. Just place the graham cracker on a plate and top it with the pudding and dollop on the whipped cream. If you would like the cracker soft, let sit for 15 minutes and enjoy.

Snack #4	Calories	Diet Snack #4	Calories
1 piece cake	600	1 fat-free brownie	100
		2 tsp. fat-free frosting	30
			130
Snack #5		**Diet Snack #5**	
5 chocolate chunk fudge cookies	500	5 fat-free choco-late fudge cookies	**250**
Snack #6		**Diet Snack #6**	
1 slice cheesecake	500	1 mini fat-free cheesecake	60
		½ C. sliced fruit	25
			85
Snack #7		**Diet Snack #7**	
1 jelly donut	350	1 English muffin	120
		2 tsp. preserves or jelly	30
			150
Snack #8		**Diet Snack #8**	
Chocolate chip ice cream sandwich	520	Diet Creamwhich: 2 fat-free chocolate chip cookies	50
		¼ C. fat-free vanilla ice cream or frozen yogurt	45
			95

You can prepare two open-faced sandwiches by simply putting half of your ice cream on each cookie, saving yourself over 400 calories!

Snack #9	Calories	Diet Snack #9	Calories
1 honey bun	475	½ bagel (frozen, small 0.75 oz.)	75
		2 tsp. Honey	30
		2 tsp. butter	66
			171
Snack #10		Diet Snack #10	
1 blueberry muffin	500	1 fat-free blueberry muffin	120

Now let's review the calorie savings of our new diet snacks.

			Calories Saved
Snack #1	vs.	Diet snack #1	460
Snack #2	vs.	Diet snack #2	250
Snack #3	vs.	Diet snack #3	365
Snack #4	vs.	Diet snack #4	470
Snack #5	vs.	Diet snack #5	250
Snack #6	vs.	Diet snack #6	415
Snack #7	vs.	Diet snack #7	200
Snack #8	vs.	Diet snack #8	425
Snack #9	vs.	Diet snack #9	304
Snack #10	vs.	Diet snack #10	380
			3,519 calories saved!

If you eat only 30 snacks per month, then you will save over 10,000 calories in one month, which in turn yields up to 36 pounds annually without subtracting volume or snacks from your diet.

CALORIE SAVING SUBSTITUTION LIST

High Calorie Item	Amount	Calories	Low calorie version	Calories	Calories saved
			Whipped Butter	70	30
			Light Butter	50	50
Butter	1 Tbsp.	100	Butter Sprinkles	15	85
			Butter Seasoning	12	88
			Butter Spray	8	92

Margarine	1 Tbsp.	100	Whipped Margarine	70	30
			Light Margarine	50	50
			Fat-Free Margarine	5	95
Mayo	1 Tbsp.	100	Light Mayonnaise	50	50
			Tofu Mayonnaise	40	60
			No Fat Mayonnaise	10	90
Oil	1 Tbsp.	120	Cooking Spray	10	110
Cream Cheese	2 Tbsp.	100	Whipped Cream Cheese	70	30
			Light Cream Cheese	50	50
			Fat Free	25	75
Sour Cream	2 Tbsp.	60	Light Sour Cream	35	25
			No-Fat Sour Cream	20	40
Heavy Cream	2 Tbsp.	120	Light Cream	60	60
			Non Dairy light	30	90
			Non Dairy Fat Free	20	100
Salad Dressing	2 Tbsp.	190	Low-cal dressing	50	140
			Fat-Free Dressing	10	180
Whipped Cream	2 Tbsp.	50	Light Whipped	15	35
			Fat-Free Whipped	5	45
Syrup, Pancake and Waffle	¼ C. (4 Tbsp.)	240	Reduced Calorie Syrup	100	140
			Light Syrup	80	160
Whole Milk	1 C.	150	2 % Milk	120	30
			1 % Milk	100	50
			Skim Milk	80	70

You can now move onto designing your own personal menu program!

9. DIET DETECTIVE

The next step on your weight loss journey is to become your own diet detective. The job of investigators is to uncover those small clues that eventually solve the whole crime. They must pay attention to detail in order to discover the clues that are left behind by the culprit. In your case, the culprit is weight gain. I'll show you the detective skills you'll need to discover how those sinister extra calories manage to "break and enter" into your diet. The weight gains that baffled you in the past won't remain unsolved mysteries for long.

Let's start by taking a discriminating look at the crime scene—where the food originated. The violation can occur in your own house or in the kitchen of your local restaurant or diner. The unknown source of your excess calories needs to be determined and reduced in order to lose weight. The only way to track the path of the caloric misconduct is to map out your eating trail. To do this establish how many times a week you eat out or consume any food prepared by someone else (e.g., relatives or friends). If you discover that your restaurant meals outnumber your home-cooked meals, then you have an obvious clue as to where the exorbitant calories are coming from. You need not be Sherlock Holmes to find this diet desperado.

REVIEWING YOUR EVIDENCE

The first step toward solving any case is to review the evidence. In this instance, your evidence is a record of what you eat and drink on a daily basis. It's time to begin writing down everything you eat and drink in your Food and Beverage Diary. If you've already been writing down your food intake, it's important to review your progress at this time. Here are important guidelines to remember when you chart your intake:

1. WRITE DOWN WHAT YOU EAT THE SAME DAY YOU EAT IT.

This is a crucial part of your program because it establishes valid documentation of what you've consumed. When a detective enters a crime scene, it's vital for them to investigate the situation as soon as possible in order to fully assess the information. The witnesses are questioned immediately while the facts are still fresh in their minds. There are two main reasons for keeping your journal up-to-date. First, it's difficult to recall everything that you eat a day or two later. I've been writing down what I eat everyday for over 20 years, and I still write it down when I eat the food. Secondly, when you add up your calories for breakfast and lunch, then you know how many calories you may allot for your snack and dinner. Your diet journal is your evidence, so please don't tamper with it or leave part of it missing from your food and beverage chart. That leads me to the second rule to follow when writing down your food intake:

2. HONESTY IS THE BEST POLICY.

It's discouraging and disheartening to add up your calories on a binge day, but it's a very crucial part of your diet program. It determines your metabolic rate and establishes a caloric reference point. If you omit certain high-calorie foods in order to reduce your total calories, then you're only cheating yourself and prolonging your weight loss program. I know this sounds rather strange to mention, but I've seen it happen over and over again. Sometimes it's a case of forgetfulness, and other times it's shame. Either way it's up to you to be honest to yourself in order to lose weight. Your food diary is a personal document, and you don't ever have to show it to anyone but yourself. If you tend to forget how many cookies you've consumed, then get out your desired portion in advance and count them because the scale still registers your "mystery calories" even if you forget to add them up.

The only way to successfully solve any case is to compile the evidence and let it lead you to the solution. As discussed previously the evidence is your diet journal. If you tamper with it, it will only taint the evidence, and then the case becomes more difficult to solve.

3. DETECT THE DIFFERENCE BETWEEN HIGH-CALORIE AND LOW-CALORIE FOOD.

It's time to take a detailed look at your diet data. The world's most prominent detectives have one thing in common, which is an eye for detail. They're able to find those little clues that everyone else overlooked. The best way to establish a dietary eye for detail is simply to determine how many calories are in each ounce. This is also called the caloric density of your food.

$$\text{Caloric Density (CD)} = \frac{\textit{Calories}}{\text{Weight of Food (in oz.)}}$$

You can see how valuable this technique is just by looking at two extreme examples:

Highest Caloric Density

Olive oil: 120 cal. per Tbsp.
(There are 2 Tbsp. in 1 oz., and olive oil has 240 cal per ounce.)

$$\text{CD} = \frac{240 \text{ cal.}}{1 \text{ oz.}} = 240 \text{ cal. per oz.}$$

Lowest Caloric Density

Lettuce: 5 net calories per 8 ounces

$$\text{CD} = \frac{5 \text{ cal.}}{8 \text{ oz.}} = .625 \text{ cal. per oz.}$$

Oil has 384 times as many calories per ounce than lettuce, which means that you can eat either 384 ounces of lettuce or only 1 ounce of olive oil. This is pure mathematics, which still doesn't take into account the fact that all the calories of olive oil are from fat and the lettuce is completely fat free. Therefore, they're certainly not equivalent in terms of nutrition.

Finer details like this can make a big difference toward your weight loss. This is fabulous news because it means that you won't have to make drastic changes in your diet in order to lose weight. Instead, you'll carefully examine the hidden calories per ounce, and that will bring your weight loss solution into full view. You can now begin to solve the mystery of your baffling weight gain!

4. REVIEW YOUR DIET JOURNAL WITH A DISCERNING EYE.

Sit down with one week's worth of your diary. Go over each individual day to determine changes you can make in order to reach your weight loss goal. Look for the items with the highest caloric density. The quickest way is to identify foods and condiments that are over 120 calories per ounce. If you think of it like a great detective—logically instead of sentimentally—then you begin to understand why you need to cut back on foods with a high caloric density.

I'll give you a perfect example. You go out to a restaurant and dessert is included, so you order a piece of pecan pie only to find that you are so stuffed from your dinner that you ask the waitress to bag it up for you to bring home. That night you put it on your food scale and realize it weighs 10 ounces. If you didn't weigh the pie, you probably would have guessed the calories for each piece based on a grocery store frozen pie, or you could have looked it up in a calorie-counting book, but the figures in such books are somewhat deceiving. This is because the portion sizes are much smaller than you're used to eating. They give the calories of an 8-inch pie, which is divided into 8 pieces. If you made this pie at home, you would normally cut it into 4 pieces. The true calories are therefore doubled! You should really count this pie as having 150 calories per ounce.

That means the dessert is 1,500 calories. Therefore, you can't just look up the lowest calorie for the smallest piece of pie in the calorie-counting book (dreaming up the calories) because you will only delay your goal, which is weight loss! So, be honest to yourself and your journal, and count your calories properly.

5. IF THE CALORIES AREN'T REVEALED BY THE LABEL, BAKERY, OR RESTAURANT, THERE'S ONE GOLDEN RULE: THE CALORIES ARE NOT LOW.

If the food's producer chose not to put their product's calorie information on the label, they're not proud of the number. If you walked into your local bakery to purchase some after-dinner desserts and you suddenly noticed that the calories were printed next to all your favorite sweets, you'd be shocked to discover that just one cookie was over 800 calories! It's comforting to imagine that the calories of the food you eat are low. This way you can keep eating the same things and blame your weight gain on something else besides your eating habits. This, however, doesn't result in weight loss. The sooner you accept that your weight is directly dependent on the net calories you consume, the sooner you can make dietary choices that result in permanent weight loss.

6. IF YOU NEED HELP STICKING TO YOUR DIET, CALL THE HELPFUL FOOD POLICE.

This is a friend with whom you share the report of your caloric details. Here's a perfect example of how police guide and improve your behavior. You're on a long vacation trip, and your children are in the backseat breathing down your neck, asking, "How long will it be before we get there?" Your lovely wife is asking you, "When can we stop and eat because everyone is hungry?" You drive faster in order to please the family. You pick up the cell phone to make reservations at the restaurant so you won't be waiting long. All of a sudden, you see a cop ahead with his radar gun pointed your way. You immediately let up on the gas, put down your cell phone, and fasten your seatbelt. Your next thought is to recall whether you brought your insurance card and if the vehicle's inspection is up-to-date. The point I'm making is simple. People react differently when they're held responsible for their actions.

This law of behavior holds true for dieting. When we know that other people are monitoring our eating habits, we tend to eat fewer calories in order to appear innocent. It's a common practice of my clients to eat less when they're in public. As one of my clients, Florence, put it, "I don't want people to taunt and tease me about going off my diet." No one in the world wants to be thought of as a failure. Another client, Starr, eats less in public because she imagines that the guests at the social events will look upon her with disgust if she binges in front of them, murmuring, "Look at that overweight woman eating those desserts. It's no wonder she looks like she does." Who knows if anyone was ever discussing her eating habits let alone her weight? Yet, the thought of what other people might think prevents her from eating "forbidden" high-calorie foods in public.

THE CASE OF THE HIDDEN CALORIE (RESTAURANT CALORIE, THAT IS.)

Your next mission as diet detective is to ask your favorite restaurants to divulge the calories of the meals you're ordering. If they don't have a clue, it's probably because they aren't concerned with the calories or don't want you to know. They prepare the food to please their customers' taste buds. Since many restaurants don't know the calories, I ask them to tell me the ingredients so I can figure out the calories myself. They usually tell me it's a secret recipe and won't give them to me.

The whole concept of going out to dinner is to leave the cooking and cleaning to someone else and enjoy the meal. Most people expect to be served large portions of rich-tasting food at a restaurant. They want to get a good deal and make it worth the price they pay. When I was a child, I still remember the buffet. My grandfather asked why I was having vegetables when there was roast beef and ham. They wanted to make sure they were getting their money's worth. Most people go to a restaurant with no intention of dieting, and they would feel cheated in a monetary sense if they had to pay high prices for a diet meal.

So first, a dieter must remember that restaurants don't go into business to serve low-calorie food. Secondly, a competitive eatery serves large portion sizes. My dieters have tried to compensate for this by bringing leftovers home and eating them the next day. This would only make sense if you eliminate a meal the next day, or else all you've done is had two high-calorie meals instead of one. The calories still entered your body whether you ate them in one day or two! Thirdly, the reason you enjoy the food so much is that the restaurant prepares it with more fat than you would ever use at home. I'll give you an example of how high in fat the average cream sauce is at a typical Italian restaurant. My dieter ordered fettuccine Alfredo with seafood and only ate half the meal. She took the rest home for lunch the next day. When she opened the refrigerator, much to her surprise, the sauce had all solidified! This indicated that it was mainly comprised of fat. Remember that each tiny teaspoon of fat is 40 calories; therefore if the sauce is eight ounces, it contains a whopping 960 calories. This is only the topping of the meal; we haven't even added the calories of the real food yet.

Another example of hidden calories comes from one of my clients who took a job at an upscale catering service. She was eating their food and gaining weight. I asked her what the chef used to prep his pasta, and she came back with the revealing answer to her suspicious weight gain. The chef was just pouring oil on all of their pasta recipes before adding any sauce. This made it easy for him because the pasta wouldn't stick together. The cook had no concept of how many calories he was pouring on; he just didn't want his pasta sticking together. Pasta is about 138 net calories per cup, but oil is 1920 calories per cup—not to mention that all the calories are derived from pure fat!

You must look at your meal through the eyes of a diet detective. Sometimes an investigator walks into a crime scene and the criminal makes it appear to be a burglary in order to cover up the real crime, which is murder. This can happen to your food. You order an "innocent" marinara sauce, which arrives at your table looking low calorie. This is only a façade because the pasta has already been prepared with oil or butter that you can't even see. Another example is the typical tossed salad. If you order it with dressing, the average cooks don't measure it. They just pour it on, and the more they give you, the more you come back. If the salad has only 100 calories and they put 4 ounces of regular dressing on it, you just topped your greens with 500 more calories.

These places make more money when they give you large portions of high-calorie food. Think about this and ask yourself if it's really worth it to pay high prices and gain weight the next day. If you really want to treat yourself, then make one of my quick gourmet diet meals and enjoy. The portion sizes of my recipes are so large that my dieters have said it takes them all week just to eat one pasta casserole.

It's your attention to detail that keeps you thin in life. The small decisions that you make every day determine what you weigh. If you really put it into perspective, it's more about the choices you make on a daily basis. You need not give up volume; you just have to give up hidden calories! If you decide you aren't willing to give up dining out, then do it less frequently. If you find yourself out at a restaurant, remember you are responsible for what you eat; don't expect the server to know what is high or low in calories. You must be aware of the mystery calories that can end up on your plate.

WHO, WHAT, WHERE, WHEN, AND WHY OF DIETING

After a few weeks on a diet, you realize that your little indulgences can add up to a lot of unnecessary calories. It's time to fine-tune your program. Fortunately, eating is a learned behavior. You can change this pattern and turn it into a weight loss behavior. First, take a look at your food and beverage recording chart and mark all of your problem areas with an asterisk. Now go over each item and ask yourself the following questions:

1. Who was I with, when I ate the excessive calories?

2. What type of food did I consume when I blew my diet?

3. Where did I eat the wrong foods?

4. When was I overeating?

5. Why did I eat the food that I shouldn't have?

Now let's go over each question in detail in order to target your specific dietary obstacles.

1. The *who* can turn out to be a long list of what I call your "binge buddies." This is the social arena where you feel free to eat what you want. When I give my clients their personal analysis test, I ask them with whom they eat breakfast, lunch, and dinner. I then ask them if these people are diet supporters or diet saboteurs. You come home at night after a long hard day at the office, and your spouse says, "Oh, honey, you shouldn't have to cook. Let's just order out Chinese." The initial response is one of habit. You think, "That sounds like a lovely idea. I've been stressed out. I deserve to relax and have my food delivered right to my door. Why should I have to prepare my own dinner?"

   Now take time out and think about your train of thought. Isn't that the way you used to rationalize your right to overeat? Don't fall back into your old pitfalls; instead train your brain to think thin. You know that when you eat restaurant food, it's high in calories and promotes the habit of eating food that's high in fat and sodium. If you repeat the behavior that led to your weight gain, the results will be the same. It's time to turn over a new dietary leaf and make a decision based upon logic, not hunger. At this point, you have two options.

   The first one is to order a diet version of Chinese food. One way this can be accomplished is to ask for steamed rice, steamed tofu, or broiled chicken without any sauce or condiment, and steamed vegetables. The key to keeping the meal low-calorie is to order it without condiments and then ask for soy sauce on the side.

   The other option is to take out a single pan and start cooking some rice or noodles, adding a low-calorie protein source such as seafood or chicken. Put a whole bag of frozen vegetables on the top just before it's finished so that the steam from the rice cooks the veggies. Then add a low-calorie condiment such as Teriyaki sauce.

Since you know you will be asked to eat out, prepare for the situation in advance. Make a list of all the people in your life who tempt you to break your diet (a chart is provided in the appendix). After each name write down whether they're normal weight or overweight. Then proceed to jot down the response you gave to each person who asked you to eat.

2. The next plan of action is to discern what food causes you to stray from your diet program. Review your diet journal and underline the highest calorie foods that contributed to the daily total yet provided little volume. Then think about why you eat those foods.

There are two main categories of junk food. They're either crunchy and salty or smooth and sweet. The crunchy group consists of foods like potato chips, tortilla chips, corn chips, etc. The smooth group includes ice cream, pudding, cake, pie, chocolate, etc. Now write down your top ten favorite selections from each group (a chart is provided in the appendix), and then choose a substitution that you can live with. See the Party Mix and Sweet Snack sections of this book to see how to exchange your high-calorie choices for low-calorie alternatives. In most cases, you only need to alter the method of preparation in order to save hundreds of calories!

A popular and healthy alternative is seasoned or spicy foods. This fusion of flavor is a dieter's friend. There are several reasons why cultures don't over-eat spicy food. The most obvious is that it leaves such a strong taste in you mouth that you don't need any more of it to satisfy you. The second reason is that it usually imparts a desire to drink water. The water in turn fills up your stomach, and you feel full. Spices also help to expedite digestion and there-fore move the food out of the system faster, thus fewer calories are absorbed. In addition, as a dieter, you benefit from spicy food because you don't need to add any fat to it. Therefore, you can subtract calories from a recipe by taking out the fat and substituting spices instead. It's a scientific fact that cultures that consume spicy foods have lower rates of obesity.

3. Your next assignment is to establish the *where* in your diet. First, take a good look at your food diary and all the foods you've underlined. Next, write down the top ten places where you overeat (a chart is provided in the appendix). The most popular locations are: workplace, parents' home,

in front of the television, surfing the Internet, and restaurants. Now, go back to the *who* list and look at the connection. Were you with these same people when you broke your diet? Is this beginning to make sense to you now? The pieces of the puzzle are fitting together to form the whole picture. The more you expose yourself to temptation, the higher the chances that you'll give in.

Once again, be prepared for these situations ahead of time. If you know that you'll be going home this evening to watch your favorite prime time TV shows, then purchase a low-calorie snack and eat that instead.

4. The next step is to determine the time of day when you tend to overeat. The most common time for dieters to overeat is in the evening, after dinner. A chart is available in the appendix to help you identify your specific eating habits.

    Once you determine the individual time frame in which you binge, you can decide the optimum plan of action. For instance, if you find yourself in front of the television with a bowl of ice cream every night between 7–9 p.m., then it's time to make some changes. You have two choices:

    *   Reduce the calories of your eating spree.

    *   Change the activity that prompts you to eat. If a certain action in your life causes an eating reaction, then change the behavior so that food isn't on your mind.

5. The next step in your dietary progress is to reveal the reasons why you overeat certain foods. This is achieved by writing down what you eat on a daily basis and thinking about the true reason for eating it. When you do this, you think of food in a whole new way. Many of my clients have told me that they stopped eating cookies because they had to count them and write them down. If you take the time to think before you eat, you'll always weigh less than the people who eat food primarily because it's there. I tell my clients to make sure it's worth the calories before you eat it, not after!

    The first important dietary "why" that needs to be discussed is why a dieter is concerned with what other people can consume. When you begin to diet, what you can and can't eat become more of an issue in your life. If you go to a party and see a skinny female eating a piece of cake, you have the tendency to think, "She can eat cake and stay slim, so why can't I? Life isn't fair; I just have a snail-like metabolism. Why not just face the facts, I'm probably doomed to be fat." This type of reasoning leads to overeating, and you should nip it in the bud.

The main thing that you should do is concentrate on your *own* progress. The person you saw eating high-calorie food might eat that way very rarely, or they might exercise for 2 hours every day. Either way, you can't let other people's eating habits influence yours. Two other factors enable other people to consume high-calorie foods. The first one is age. They may be twenty years younger than you, but by the time they get to your age, they will probably be overweight based upon pure mathematics. Secondly, they could be eating so much that they're on their way up (the weight gaining stage). Think of how much you were eating while you were gaining weight. You also can't expect the whole world to be on a diet just because you are. You need to stay focused and remember that you probably had the liberty to eat whatever you wanted for plenty of years. Now is the time to take responsibility for your actions and do something to reverse your weight gain.

My own personal reason for choosing certain foods is primarily based on taste and volume. I want my food to please my palate and fill my stomach. Then I have to think about nutritional needs as well, so I plan every supper by having a carbohydrate, a protein, and a cooked and/or raw vegetable.

The reason people overeat is based on several criteria. Food is first registered in our brain by its scent. This is so important to appetite that grocery stores across America installed bakeries in a strategic position in order to promote sales. They are often right next to the shopping carts. This way, the innocent shopper comes in to purchase a couple of items and smells the baking bread, and all of the sudden their sensory neurons take over and they feel hungry, which in turn prompts them to purchase more groceries.

The important part of the *why* in eating is to become consciously aware of your unconscious food cravings. Let's take an intricate look at what actually happens to your mind before you even take the first bite. First, we smell the food and establish a memory attached to the scent. It's important to remember that eating habits are a learned behavior. We tend to eat the foods that recreate a memory. A perfect example is cake. When you visualize cake, you're reliving a yearly memory, one that's so engraved in your brain that it almost becomes an automatic response. The first birthday party is always a gala event. How many times have you seen pictures or videos of yourself with frosting and cake smeared on your face while destroying your first piece of cake? You celebrate another year of living with this symbol–every year the same thing over and over again. Have you ever attended a birthday or wedding without cake? The food becomes a representation of the event. You remember what it tastes like before you even take your first bite of it, but if you look at food for what it signifies, then your brain is in control instead of your stomach.

Now that we've established that food is first recognized by scent then sight and then memory, the question is: when we eat a specific food, are we taking a walk down memory lane, or are we establishing a new mental image? That is, are we mindlessly repeating the mistakes of the past, or are we creating smart new habits of success?

The next step in the why process occurs after the first taste of food. This is the point where your taste buds take advantage of the situation. Your brain is bypassed as your taste buds instruct your body to continue or stop based on your individual food preferences. Don't let your taste buds become the decision makers! The flavor of the first bite convinces you that the entire snack will be equally tasty, but it won't be. I have always told my clients that the first bite is the best, and the rest is the rest. You must realize this before you over-indulge, and keep your brain in control. If you take time to think about what you're going to consume before you eat it, you'll be better off and don't waste time obsessing about what you can't have. This leads to a pity party and often results in binging. These are the thoughts that go through the human mind even before a single bite is eaten.

There are many factors that affect why we eat the foods we do. Each person has a reason that's unique to their specific food memory. You know that as a child most of us ate without a care in the world. We devoured a cookie or cupcake without the thought of its consequences. This carefree method of eating continued until we gained weight. Then food was looked upon as our enemy instead of a friend and comforter. So now, we must learn to eat like an adult. You have to decide between one food or another, because eating everything and anything you want is no longer an option. If you've been consuming food without responsibility, then it takes time for you to adjust to your new limitations. You must now try to eat with your conscience instead of with your eyes.

Now take the time to write a list of your top ten danger foods. You can use the chart provided in the appendix. Next, you'll write down the actual reason you desire this specific food. This gets to the heart of your danger foods. I ask my clients to write down the five foods they cannot live with-out, and none of them have been nutritious low-calorie foods. If they were, then they wouldn't have been coming to me to lose weight.

Now that you've determined your favorite foods, it's time to take a list and jot down the calories. Take a good look at this and think about it! Ask yourself if these foods are worth the calories. Then make a list of substitutions that will lower your caloric intake. For instance, if you feel that you cannot live without pizza, then take the time to buy pizza dough without any added oil and prepare a gourmet diet pizza. Now you can enjoy your forbidden food without any guilt or weight gain.

If you're not willing to lower the calories of the danger foods, then you must be prepared to eat smaller portions of them in order to reduce the calories. This is not an advisable method, since most of my dieters say that once they take the first bite, they often find themselves eating much more of these foods than they planned to. *If you can't control the reaction, then don't start the action!*

Finally, the most important dieting "why" is to personally determine why you'll be making wiser food choices. You need to look ahead and visualize what's going to happen to your life. It's not about a number on a scale. It's about the way you feel when you get yourself ready in the morning to face the world. One client put it into perspective when she described her own reason why she decided to lose weight. With a look of desperation in her eyes, she told me that she didn't want to look at her own body anymore. Another client told me that whenever she was at a social event and started eating, she thought that the normal-weight people in the room were all looking at her and thinking, *why is that fat lady eating so much?*

10. CARBOHYDRATES ON TRIAL

OPENING STATEMENT

The latest trend of the diet industry is to falsely attack the carbohydrate. *Low-carb foods have become too much of an obsession, and this is unwise.* Carbs are one of the six nutrients required to sustain life. Without them you would deteriorate and perish. The latest method of unhealthy dieting has been resurrected from the year 1864. The book *The Drinking Man's Diet* was written by a casket maker, oddly enough, and also condoned the daily consumption of alcohol. Then a man in 1961 tried to publish another book on this topic and was sent to jail for fraud.

The diet industry then realized that the government was not going to tolerate these lies anymore.

It wasn't until 1991 that another book was published promoting a high-protein diet; this time the author had plenty of money to promote his concept. The country became bombarded with ad after ad telling the consumer it was the diet to be on. The problem with a diet that promotes poor eating habits is that it results in permanent health problems. Every leading scientist in the field of diet and nutrition agrees that you need a balanced diet consisting of whole grains, fruits, and vegetables in order to live a long and fruitful life.

I know that dieting itself is difficult enough, so why limit your volume by eliminating the foods that fill you up? The perfect way to avoid hunger is to eat plenty of rice, pasta, potatoes, and breads (whole grains are the best for your net calories). You can't live on a program that expects you to fill up on protein and fat. An excess of protein causes a uric acid build-up in your bloodstream, which can lead to arthritis and gout. The consumption of a high-protein diet also leads to kidney and liver damage that is irreversible. There is no need to punish your body physically by eliminating a food group, nor should you pay extremely high prices for pseudo food that doesn't taste like what it's supposed to.

New age sweeteners have names that are 50–60 letters long and have no long-term studies done to determine their side effects or their safety. Remember that the food industry told us saccharin was safe when it first hit the grocery store shelves, and we know how grim that story ends. These so-called low-carb foods also use glycerin in order to cut down on the carb content. This is a product used by the natural foods industry to make soap. That's why most of the bars taste so similar to soap; they're comprised of the same ingredient.

I used the phrase "so-called low carb" because the FDA does not regulate the labels at the present time. The FDA demanded that they stop all terms like net carb, net impact carb, effective carb, and all other terms that distort the real carbohydrate value listed on the label. The companies received warning letters and were told they would have to pay fines for breaking the law. The companies knew that their only selling point was to deceive the customer into thinking that their products were low carb, when they were not, according to the nutrition facts label. The only way they could continue to make millions of dollars was by lying on their labels, so they decided to pay their fines rather than become a legitimate company, or shall I say a bankrupt one. The FDA requires all low-carb foods to put this on their label: "This is not a reduced-calorie food." And the new law for diet claims also requires them to say in their ads, "when used in conjunction with a low-calorie diet and regular exercise." The public has a right to know what goes on behind the scenes in order to make a logical decision.

Another problem with this type of low-carb food is the fat and calorie content. Companies have come out with low-carb tortilla chips that have more fat and calories than the regular ones they make. How can a food be called diet and have more calories? That makes no dietary or common sense at all. It's just a massive money-making scheme, not a diet! With the right marketing campaign, you can sell anything. Think of it; people even bought the pet rock at one point and time. When the low-carb diet came out again, I called it "the cubic zirconium of diets set in fool's gold!" I also coined it the George Orwellian diet! It just upsets me when an innocent dieter gets misled.

In my defense of the all-important carbohydrate, let me point out that cultures that have the highest intake of them have the lowest rate of obesity. Countries that exist primarily on rice, beans, corn, and yams are very thin. Yes, all the carbohydrates they can consume, and they have the lowest rate of cancer, heart disease, and obesity.

Let's look at the bodybuilder to help provide a useful example. In order to gain weight, they increase their intake of protein. They must also stay lean in order to show off their well-developed muscles. The body builder does this by eating a very low-fat, high-carbohydrate diet. The only time they will ever go low carb is for 2–4 days before a competition. You can only deprive yourself of carbohydrates for a short period of time because any longer will result in electrolyte imbalances and potassium loss, which increase your risk of a heart attack. Yes, it's that dangerous. You're basically flirting with disaster. The only reason they eat this low-carbohydrate diet is to lose water weight, plain and simple; that's all you will lose if you're eating the same calories!

The other frightening aspect of this diet is ketosis. The true meaning of this term is the discharge of toxins into the bloodstream before death or starvation. Nurses have told me they can smell ketosis on someone's breath right before they pass away. The body is an intricate piece of machinery, and you should not upset its chemical equilibrium just to lose a couple pounds of water.

The major stumbling block is that when you count only carbs, you're adding up only part of the total. A perfect analogy is your bank account. Think of your balance as the total calories you have consumed, and each check going in and out has to be counted so you won't become overdrawn. If you only counted the checks ending in even numbers, you would soon find letters in your mailbox for overdrawn checks. You will have the same problem with the scale if you try to count only the carb portion of your total food intake. The scale doesn't forget the calories from all the protein, carbs, and fats you have eaten, and you'll soon recognize the proof when you step on and see the weight gain. In terms of mathematics, it makes no logical sense to count part of the total.

Let's look at this in terms of label science. On the food label, the total calories are derived by summing up the calories from carbs, fats, and proteins.

A sample label is as follows:

Calories 156

Carbohydrates 23 g

Protein 7 g

Fat 4 g

There are 4 calories per gram of carbohydrate.
There are 4 calories per gram of protein.
There are 9 calories per gram of fat.

Carbs: 23 g x 4 = 92 calories

Protein: 7 g x 4 = 28 calories

Fat: 4 g x 9 = *36 calories*
_____

Total calories 156 calories

You can see that carbs aren't the only factor needing to be counted. If the fat and protein rise, so will the total calories: TC = Carbs + Fat + Protein

Those who reduce carbohydrate consumption may end up replacing it with more protein and fats. Why replace something that is 4 calories per gram with another thing (fat) that's 9 calories per gram? That would double your calories and half your volume. This would result in dietary sabotage. This proves that real weight loss can only be accomplished by keeping track of the number that really determines your weight loss: the total net calories that you absorb!

DIET COURT

Let's take an in-depth look at each of the accused.

"THE FIRST CARB I WILL CALL TO THE STAND IS THE POTATO."

Diet Court: Could you please state your full name and calories?

Answer: I am a potato. My proper name is Solanum Tuberosum, and I come in several varieties, shapes, and forms, such as Russet, Blue and Yukon gold. I only contain 120 net calories per cup and contain 600 mg of potassium, as well as many essential minerals.

Diet Court: How much fat do you have per cup?

Answer: None!

Diet Court: Then could you explain to the jury how you were falsely charged with impeding weight loss?

Answer: It isn't the potato that's the issue; it's what our culture does to it. Over 60 percent of the potato crop in America is used to make french fries and potato chips. The calories then soar to 150 per ounce verses 15 calories per ounce for the plain potato. Take a look at a bag of regular potato chips; the calories are 150 x 8 ounces for a total of 1,200 calories. The calories from the potato are only 500. The rest of the calories are from the oil they were fried in.

Diet Court: What is the problem with a baked potato?

Answer: The problem with the potato is the condiments. An average baked potato is only 90 calories. Now put on 2 tablespoons butter, which is 240 calories, and 2 tablespoons sour cream, which is 120 calories, for a total of 450 calories. The potato is 90 of the 450, which is only 20 percent of the total calories! Any food can be adulterated and put into a high-calorie form. Then why blame the food that contributes the least amount of calories to the total? It makes no sense at all. In closing, I would like to say: a potato a day keeps obesity away.

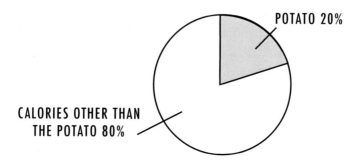

POTATO 20%

CALORIES OTHER THAN
THE POTATO 80%

"THE NEXT CARB I CALL TO THE STAND IS PASTA."

Diet Court: Could you please state your full name and calories?

Answer: I am pasta from the genus Triticum and grown as annual cereal grass. I come in several grain variations such as whole wheat, kamut, quinoa, and spelt and can be molded into various shapes and forms. I only contain an average of 120 net calories per cup when cooked.

Diet Court: How much fat do you have?

Answer: None!

Diet Court: Could you illustrate to the jury how you were under attack by suspicious diet plans?

Answer: The reason that pasta took a bad rap is the toppings, not what's underneath. The most commonly used condiments are meatballs and tomato sauce. The average meatball contains 200 calories. If you use oil to prevent it from sticking together, a half-cup will add a whopping 960 calories to your recipe! The typical Alfredo sauce is comprised of butter, cream, and parmesan cheese. This tops the calorie charts at over 1,000 calories per cup. A 4-ounce serving of pasta is only 240 net calories, which is a caloric bargain for the volume you receive. The predominant portion of the calories in a pasta meal comes from the protein and condiments. You can't take a food that's only 240 calories and pour on 1,200 calories, which now adds up to

1,440 calories. The calories from the pasta are only 17 percent of the total calories. If anything is to blame, it's the other 83 percent of the calories.

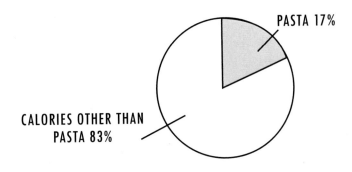

"THE NEXT CARB I CALL TO THE STAND IS RICE."

Diet Court: Could you please state your full name and calories?

Answer: My name is rice; my botanical name is Oryza Sativa, which is a cereal grass. The part of me that is actually consumed is the seed. I come in several hundred varieties, and I only contain an average of 135 net calories per cup.

Diet Court: How much fat do you contain?

Answer: None!

Diet Court: Could you please explain to the jury the unjustifiable accusations you have recently dealt with?

Answer: Rice is a staple food in the world's largest countries. The most common methods of consumption in the United States include the pork-fried variety served at a typical fast-food Chinese Restaurant. Take a good look at the cardboard container that they give you to take it home in. Let it sit for an hour and look at the box. It has oil stains seeping out of it; this is not a good sign. The calories from oil are 120 per tablespoons. If the typical cup of fried rice contains even 4 tablespoons, there are 480 calories from oil! Now let's examine the protein in this dish. Pork has 100 calories per ounce, so even if there are only 2 ounces in the rice, this adds 200 more calories to the total. The total calories are now 135 from rice, 480 from fat, and 200 from pork, which equals 815 calories. The rice contributed only 16 percent of the total calories.

The second garden-variety rice dish is the pilaf. The conventional method of preparation is butter. An average serving can contain up to 4 tablespoons of fat. So there are 135 net calories in the cup of rice, plus 480 calories in the butter, for a total of 615 calories. The rice only supplies 22 percent of the total calories of the recipe.

The third traditional rice dish is Spanish rice. This is usually comprised of rice, tomato sauce, and ground beef. Some ready-made pasta sauces can be as high as 300 calories per cup. If the protein is run-of-the-mill ground beef, it's 100 calories per ounce. Therefore, an average serving of Spanish rice will have 1 cup of rice at 135 calories, a half-cup of sauce at 150 calories, and a half-cup of beef at 400 calories—a total of 685 calories. The rice is responsible for only 135 of the 685, which is only 20 percent of the recipe. Mathematically speaking, it is impossible to blame the lowest calorie item in any recipe! So, go ahead and enjoy, because rice is nice!

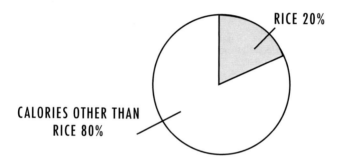

RICE 20%

CALORIES OTHER THAN
RICE 80%

"THE NEXT CARB I CALL TO THE STAND IS GRAINS."

Diet Court: Could you please state your full name and calories?

Answer: I am commonly referred to as the staff of life and come in several varieties including whole wheat, rye, corn, raisin, sourdough, pumpernickel, French, and Italian. I am approximately 50 net calories per ounce

Diet Court: How much fat do you contain?

Answer: None!

Diet Court: Now it's time for you to rise up to the occasion and expose the truth about bread and grain products. Could you clarify to the public why grains were incriminated by some skeptics?

Answer: Many Americans start the day with bakery products, such as donuts. Let's take the glazed donut as an example. The total calories are 350. The label reads as follows:

Calories 350
Fat 19 g
Carbs 41 g
Sugars 21 g
Protein 4 g

To determine the actual percent of calories from the grain, we must subtract out the rest of the calories as follows:

Fat: 19 g x (9 cal. per gram) = 171 calories
Sugars: 21 g x (4 cal. per g) = 84 calories
Protein: 4 g x (4 cal. per g) = 16 calories

Now that we have transformed the grams into calories, we can subtract them from the total count.

350 calories
- 171 cal from fat
-84 cal from sugar
-16 cal from protein
79 calories from flour

The actual percent of calories from the flour is 79 of the 350, which equals 22 percent of the total calories. This once again proves that the grain (flour) is only one-fifth of the total calories of the donut.

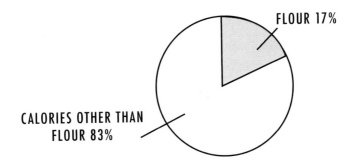

FLOUR 17%

CALORIES OTHER THAN
FLOUR 83%

"THE NEXT CARB I CALL TO THE STAND IS THE MUFFIN."

Diet Court: Could you explain the problem with muffins?

Answer: It sounds like a healthy way to start the day until we take a closer, more discerning look at the calories. The average restaurant or grocery store muffin contains approximately 650 calories. After subtracting the calories from the fat, sugar, and protein, as described above, the percent of calories from the flour is only 24% of the total calories.

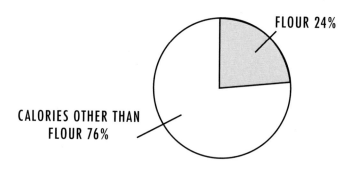

FLOUR 24%

CALORIES OTHER THAN
FLOUR 76%

"THE NEXT CARB I CALL TO THE STAND IS FRUIT."

Diet Court: Could you please state your full name and average calories?

Answer: I come in many varieties, shapes, and forms and grow in different climates around the globe. My average calories are 50 per cup.

Diet Court: Do you contain any fat?

Answer: None!

Diet Court: Please give the jury a description of the obstacles you have faced in your recent attack.

Answer: When dieters go on an all-fruit diet for one week, they will lose as much as 10 pounds during that time. It is the perfect food for a dieter, because it fills you up and provides numerous micronutrients as well as vitamin C. The problem with fruit is the preparation. If you put me in a pie, for example, the calories will soar from 50 to 500. The actual calories coming from fruit are only 10 percent of the total calories. Once again, it's the way you consume

11. GET RAW

The whole concept of eating raw food in order to encourage weight loss has become a trendy dietary phenomenon. There are several books that hail the praises of eating a raw food diet. It's obvious that raw food supplies the body with enormous health benefits, but most programs are rather restrictive and therefore short-lived. The logical conclusion is therefore to incorporate raw food into your diet in a manner that fits your own style. When my clients ask me if they must eat raw food to lose weight, I respond: *"You don't have to do anything you don't want to on my program."* I will give you the facts and let you decide for yourself how raw food will fit into your diet plan. Here are just a few vital reasons to eat raw food daily:

1. *Your body will receive the full benefits of each micronutrient the food contains.* This is because the chemical composition of the food isn't altered, and therefore the nutrients are "bioavailable." The dieter feels satisfied because the nutrients quell his or her hunger.

2. *It's often high in fiber.* This helps to move food and calories through the digestive tract quicker, which in turn reduces the rate of caloric absorption. The result is simple yet brilliant: the fewer calories you absorb, the less you weigh! It's similar to getting a bonus in your paycheck. In this case, you get caloric rewards with minimal effort.

3. *The body is supplied with enzymes.* Enzymes are essential for all food digestion, absorption, and metabolism in the human body. They're the catalysts that allow us to utilize the nutrients in our food. They speed up the process of digestion. When the body is deprived of enzymes because we don't consume raw food or take enzyme supplements, the body must resort to using up its own digestive enzymes. This depletes the body of its own reserve, which in turn results in poor digestion and a weakened immune system. The eventual outcome of a deficiency of enzymes is a lack of energy. In time it can lead to the development of degenerative diseases such as arthritis, cancer, and circulatory disorders, so the importance of ingesting an ample supply of enzymes should not be taken lightly. The most notable

reward from increasing your enzyme supply is the boosting of your energy level. It's commonplace to hear overweight individuals complain of a lack of energy. This is primarily a result of poor eating habits that eventually leads to low enzyme levels.

Treating food with pesticides, herbicides, and fungicides depletes the enzyme content of food, as does the manner in which our food is processed, frozen, heated, cooked, and microwaved. The solution is to try to eat some raw food daily and take my digestive enzyme with your meals that I have designed specifically for dieters. This supplement is discussed in detail in the section entitled Dieter's Little Helper.

Now let's examine how raw food enhances your weight loss program. The best advantage is that you get the most volume for the least amount of calories. In other words, raw foods have a low caloric density. By weight, the main constituent of raw fruits and vegetables is water. The high H_2O content provides lots of volume, which helps you feel full, and these foods tend to satisfy both your hunger and thirst simultaneously! A perfect example comes to mind. It's a hot, humid, summer day and you see a ripe watermelon at the local farmers market. The mere sight of it invokes pleasant childhood memories. Then before you know it, your salivary glands begin to anticipate the succulent sweetness of your first bite. It's too late to turn back now, and soon the precious melon is cradled in your arms. As you drive home, you begin to contemplate whether you want to wait for it to chill in the refrigerator or bring it out to the picnic table and eat a slice as you enjoy the pleasantries of a summer afternoon. There is no group of foods on earth that can fill you up without filling you out like raw fruits and vegetables.

Another benefit of enjoying uncooked food is that it requires more chewing, so you tend to eat at a slower pace. This is always a benefit to dieters, because the slower you eat, the less you eat. The reason is that the brain needs 10–20 minutes to sense that you're full, so after your stomach has truly had enough, you could keep eating for another 10 minutes before your brain finally gets the message. Think of all the wasted calories! When you eat slowly, your brain has more time to keep pace with your stomach, so you stop eating when you're really full. That's why it's undeniably beneficial to include raw food in your diet. Slow down your meals, and you'll speed up your weight loss.

Once I discovered that raw food facilitates weight loss, the next step was to discover how to eat them on a daily basis. The simple rule of thumb I give my diet clients is to eat at least one raw food each day. The first step is to write down a list of your favorite fruits and vegetables.

If you don't feel like making a list at the moment, you can refer to the chapter titled Easy Net Calorie Charts. There's a list of fruits and vegetables with their corresponding net calorie values already calculated for your convenience. It's actually the preferable method because it lists dozens of fruits and vegetables so that you can compare their net calorie values. It also enables you to refresh yourself and choose options you might have otherwise overlooked. It's always advantageous to expand your food horizons in order to enhance weight loss.

Now that you know the benefits of having raw food daily, I'll show you several ways you can effortlessly include them in your meals and snacks.

OPTIMUM WAYS TO SNEAK RAW FOOD INTO YOUR DIET

1. Start off the day with the energy of raw food.

    When you begin adding raw food to your breakfast, you'll feel more energized and satisfied than you can imagine.

    A. Add chopped fresh fruit to your hot or cold cereal.

    B. When eating a bread product such as toast, bagels, or English muffins, try using Neufchatel cheese and fresh fruit as a condiment.

    C. If you prefer low-calorie yogurt, add some extra fresh fruit, because the fruit inside isn't raw.

    D. When making omelets, don't cook the vegetables. You can melt a bit of gourmet cheese inside, and then top it off later with raw diced onions, peppers, and mushrooms. Use your imagination. The omelet can also be adorned with chopped fresh fruit, if you prefer.

    E. When you prepare waffles, top them with fresh fruit and real maple syrup or raw honey.

    F. If you should cook pancakes, don't put the fruit into the batter. It's better to add your blueberries or other fruit on top of the flapjacks. This allows you to savor the flavor and enjoy the benefits of raw food simultaneously.

2. It's time to experience a real power lunch.

    A. This is a perfect time of day to sit down to a vegetable salad. The key here is to avoid the pitfalls of hidden calories. It's best if you eliminate meat and oil from the salad because the calories tend to add up much too quickly. Why waste 120 precious calories on only 3 teaspoons of oil? It's simply not worth it. A dieter should conserve their calories for food, not condiments. The best salad dressing is a low-calorie one. The beauty of having a salad for lunch is that the variety and volume make a perfect duo for fulfillment. It's always enjoyable to munch on a fresh salad made from fresh seasonal vegetables based upon your own personal choices. I advise my clients to try a new vegetable, or one they haven't eaten in a while, on a weekly basis. This gives the taste buds something to look forward to.

B. If you normally pack a sandwich for lunch, then use your bread as a template for raw veggies. It's always advantageous for a dieter to break the sandwich rules. The average run-of-the-mill sandwich involves mustard or mayonnaise, a couple of pieces of lunchmeat, and a slice of cheese. It all seems innocent until you add up the calories. The volume isn't sufficient to warrant the caloric content. The best way to prepare a sandwich is open faced. The primary reason for doing this is that it allows you to stack your vegetables on top of your bread. It also takes more time to eat two open-faced sandwiches with vegetables than it does a plain luncheon meat sandwich. The typical choices for vegetables include lettuce, tomato, onion, and sprouts. It's important that you use a low-calorie condiment on your recipe.

C. If you're in a hurry and don't have time to prepare a low-calorie lunch, you can grab a pita with some cucumber, tomato, cheese, and a bottle of low-calorie dressing for a quick midday meal. The options for vegetable selections are completely up to you. Your choice of bread products should be based on their caloric and fiber content. This in turn will lower the net calorie content of your lunch.

D. If you prefer to eat fruit for lunch, then make yourself a delicious fresh fruit salad. The high water content of the fruit keeps you satisfied until dinner. The volume also keeps your stomach full.

3. Dinner is another perfect meal for including raw foods.

A. It's time to spice up your night with Mexican cuisine. The obvious choice that includes raw food is the versatile taco. The taco shell should be soft and baked in order to conserve calories. There are some companies that make a low-calorie hard shell, which is suitable if they're warmed in the oven and not fried in oil. The protein selections are based on your own personal choices, but be looking for proteins with fewer calories per ounce. For instance, if you like both chicken and beef, it's favorable to choose chicken's 50 calories per ounce versus beef, which can be up to 100 calories per ounce. The next step is to prepare your taco bar. This buffet approach enables the dieting members of the family to choose the lower-calorie toppings. That way you can enjoy a wholesome meal without sacrificing volume or taste. The taco bar is built by arranging your favorite chopped vegetables in bowls, ready to be served. The traditional choices are onions, green, yellow and/or red peppers, and lettuce. The cheese should be shredded and served at room temperature in order to savor its flavor. If you decide to top your taco with sour cream, do make sure it's low calorie. The lowest-calorie condiment for your recipe is salsa. You can choose from various types, but the market now offers gourmet selections, which turn an ordinary Mexican meal into an extraordinary one. (If you want to give your taste buds a real treat, try a pineapple salsa.) You should assemble each of your toppings in individual bowls and let members of the family prepare their tacos according to their own caloric allotment.

B. You can also transform your kitchen into a salad bar. The entire family will enjoy taking part in preparing the quick salad recipes. Besides the garden style, two other options are the potato salad or pasta salad. The idea is to incorporate raw food into the meal. The raw item selections should be chopped, diced, or sliced and put into separate containers. Then arrange your toppings on the table or counter so that each family member can build his or her own unique salad. Following is a list of raw salad suggestions:

Raw Vegetables	Amt	Net Calories
Asparagus tips	1 C.	30
Bamboo Shoots	1 C.	30
Broccoli Florets	1 C.	20
Cabbage, green	1 C.	5
Cabbage, red	1 C.	5
Carrots	1 C.	30
Cauliflower	1 C.	15
Celery	1 C.	2
Green beans	1 C.	30
Lettuce	1 C.	5

Mung bean sprouts	1 C.	10
Mushrooms	1 C.	14
Onions	1 C.	40
Peas, sugar snap	1 C.	45
Peppers, sweet	1 C.	14
Radishes	1 C.	5
Sauerkraut	1 C.	20
Spinach	1 C.	5
Squash, summer	1 C.	10
Tomato	1 C.	20

The conventional condiment for potato or pasta salad is regular mayonnaise. This is not a "diet friendly" dressing because it has 100 calories per tablespoon. The preferred alternative is low calorie mayonnaise or diet salad dressing. This decreases the calories and increases the flavor. The precise directions and recipes are included in the section of this book titled "Quick Salad Ideas."

4. If you decide to snack, do it intelligently.

The conventional snack usually involves "munching out" on high-calorie junk foods. The consequences are often calorie overload. The dieter ends up consuming so many calories that they can't lose weight. This usually leaves the dieter in a delicate state of mind. The doubts begin to swirl in the mind: "To diet or not to diet, that is the question." The purpose of a snack is not to sabotage your diet.

To use the analogy of a concert, think of the snack as the warm-up band. It gets you in the mood for the headliner band, which in this case repre-sents your meal. I prefer to call it an appetizer instead of a snack. The new sophisticated terminology imparts a vision of gourmet cheese, a fresh fruit, and imported olives versus potato chips and dip. When you look at a snack as a special treat instead of a binge, you'll make better food choices. The snack is an opportune time to eat raw food.

My experience with snacking changed when I realized how many calories I was wasting by eating calorically dense food. The concept of eating raw food instead of traditional munchies came about as a result of attending art receptions. The galleries usually provide a buffet of food for their potential customers. The items varied according to the budget of each venue. The typical fare consisted of cheese, crackers, a vegetable platter, fruit platter, and assorted desserts. The art galleries usually coordinate their openings together, and therefore you can attend over ten receptions in one evening. This habit can lead to weight gain if you're not "calorie wise." I always tell my clients, "You need to plan in advance for social events." If you know you'll be eating out that evening, then reduce your calorie intake during the day. This allows you to bank up your calories for later. It's comforting to tell yourself you won't be eating that much, but when you get home afterward and start adding up the calories, the damage is already done. The logical way to handle social gatherings without weight gain is to eat fewer calories before the event so that you give yourself some caloric leeway.

The optimum way to incorporate raw food with your snack is to use fruits and vegetables in a creative way. I'll give you a perfect example. I decided that when I wanted to eat a piece of cheese, the cracker under it wasn't worth the calories. Your basic run-of-the-mill cracker just sort of melts in your mouth and gets in-between your teeth. I was looking for a substitute, and cucumber slices worked perfectly. The vegetable provided more crunch and flavor than the disintegrating cracker. Another item I substituted for a cracker was a julienne strip of red pepper. It was a pleasant surprise as my taste buds enjoyed the succulent combination of the juicy pepper and the tangy piece of Brie cheese that accompanied it. The vegetable platter is diet friendly, but the dip that usually sits in the center of the innocent vegetables is diet unfriendly. The average conventional dip usually contains 70–100 calories per tablespoon. I've observed the eating habits of other people for over twenty years, and the average dipper uses at least a tablespoon each time they dip. You can eat a whole cup of cucumber slices for 14 net calories. If you douse each slice with dip, the calorie damage will go from 14 to 1,014 calories! It's best to forego the dip and eat a couple of gourmet pieces of cheese instead.

The fruit platter provides ample opportunity to enjoy raw food. I usually opt for grapes because they satisfy my desire for something sweet and juicy. They're only 40 net calories per cup, and they're ranked third on the satisfaction list. A fruit platter is a perfect way to sneak some raw food and enjoy yourself simultaneously.

When you're snacking at home, let your own preferences guide you, or if you're preparing a snack for the family, the choices should be agreed upon in advance.

A. You can make up a fruit salad or fruit platter in advance so it's ready for evening snacking. There are plenty of low-calorie condiments available for your dip, ranging from whipped cream to low-calorie flavored yogurts.

B. If you prefer vegetables, then prepare a vegetable plate and store it in your refrigerator so it's available for your snacking pleasure. There are many low-calorie dressings and diet sour cream dips that can adorn your vegetables.

It's evident that consuming raw food as part of your diet program encourages weight loss. The health benefits of eating raw food are an added bonus. The moral of the story is: once you begin eating raw food on a daily basis, you'll be *in awe of raw!*

12. THE TIMELINE OF HUNGER

Did you ever wonder how it all got out of control? Why does man find himself reaching for his second bowl of ice cream when the first one was enough? How come one cookie isn't adequate, and we find ourselves with an empty box by the end of the evening? Why are we hungry even when our body doesn't need the calories? How come a person that is 50 pounds overweight needs to keep eating more and more to stay satisfied?

The only way to solve a problem is to start at the beginning and work your way toward the solution. It all started in a perfect place called the Garden of Eden, which you could say we turned into the Garden of Evil, when man had to go out every day in order to gather his food. The mere act of obtaining your food from nature burns calories. If you actually had to perform physical labor in order to acquire your daily food allotment, I'll bet you would think twice about eating it all in one big binge!

In the little house on the prairie days, food was looked upon in a different manner. You cleared your land, then you planted your crops, prayed for a good growing season, and tended to your crop for months before you even thought about being able to eat the food. Then came the fruition of your farming, and the family would anticipate the coming of the crop. A time of harvest is a time of joy! Think about the amount of time and effort that went into each and every bit of food they obtained.

In the event of a great growing season, the work was not finished yet. The family then had to gather the crop and prepare it for storage. In order to prepare the family dinner, you had to cut down a tree, dry the wood, and then start a fire. This was all done before you even got to eat your first morsel of food. Now I understand the importance of saying grace before eating. The culture was thankful to the Lord for providing them with a bountiful crop so that they could nourish themselves.

Now let's fast forward to the era of modern agriculture. As soon as food became a moneymaking commodity, the whole world changed. Now the goal was to produce more crops for less money. It wasn't about growing food to feed your family. The farmer then wanted to protect his crop because it was his livelihood. If he could yield more produce, he would make more money. One way he could do this was by protecting the crops. This was first accomplished with great success by natural means until the invention of the pesticide. These corporations then convinced the innocent and sometimes less educated farmer that this was the proper thing to do. The first back draft was cancer. Conventional farmers have the highest cancer rates in the world. Then came nature's recourse. The pesky little plant predators became resistant to the poisons and eventually ate their crops anyway. New types of pestilence were showing up all over the globe. This chemical laden food also had another less noticeable problem. It contains less vitamins and minerals. Which means the people would have to eat more food in order to obtain their essential nutrients. The public will have to eat more in order to satisfy their hunger. Well, that didn't bother the farmer. *If people need to eat more, we sell more!*

The next step in agricultural progress was to prolong the shelf life of food. If scientists could prevent spoilage, the losses would be less for the vendors, i.e., grocery stores. This was accomplished with the invention of preservatives. This sounded like a fine idea because the increased shelf life provided more of an opportunity to sell the product. The chemicals were listed on the ingredients as letters, so the public didn't pay much attention to them. BHA and BHT sound simple enough, yet if these chemicals are listed by their proper names, you start to wonder what are you really putting into your body. The precise names of two preservatives are Butylated Hydroxyanisole and Butylated Hydroxytoluene. The average consumer doesn't even know what they are eating anymore. These preservatives are known to cause health-related problems. The addition of preservatives to food decreased the consumption of fresh food, which is essential to good health and longevity. An increased shelf life also means a decreased nutrient value.

The entrepreneurs were at it again; they decided to enhance the flavor of food. This way you would purchase more of it, and the food giants would in turn make more money. The goal was to produce the food in a more cost effective manner. In engineering terms, we call it optimization. In terms of your health, we call it devastation. The origination of artificial colors and flavors was on the horizon. Food would then be more visually appealing. The cost of production would decrease, and thus the profit margin would increase. The only problem was food would never be the same again. Scientists admit that when a label states artificial flavors, it can contain 100 different chemicals to lure you into overeating. They in turn describe the combination of these chemicals as a drug like affect on the human body. This means that food could be as addicting as drugs and tobacco. You won't just be satisfied with one cookie anymore; now you'll eat the whole bag. This works out perfectly for the food company because they will increase their sales and in turn profits. The type of food you choose to eat determines whether you will feel hungry or full when you are done eating! If you can't pronounce or understand the ingredients in your food, don't eat it.

Food science began to progress at an amazing pace. With the increase in food technology came an increase in hunger. The next step mankind made was to invent the concept of fast-food restaurants. A place for the public to breeze in and leave with food in hand, or should I say with calories in hand. Where else can you go in the world to purchase 5,000 calories for less than five dollars? Let me point out that every time we start a fast-food chain in a country that never had such a restaurant, the obesity rates soar! The idea is good for the owner but not for the poor consumer. The customers often gobble up their purchase at the location or while driving home from the eatery. That's not conducive to dieting because you consume too many calories in too short a time. You don't obtain enough nutrients or volume to stay satisfied, and you find yourself looking for something more to munch upon. When fast-food restaurants first opened in the United States, it was a once-a-week visit that was considered a treat. When you consider the unhealthy side effects, it's not really a treat at all; it's more like a punishment. You cannot consume your daily caloric allotment in one meal and expect to maintain your weight, let alone lose weight. It's not worth the temptation. I don't want to go there and eat a salad with low-calorie dressing and watch everyone else eating burgers and fries and milkshakes. The goal is not to punish yourself. You should pamper yourself.

In man's never-ending quest for new restaurant schemes, came the all-you-can-eat buffet. The public adored the concept. Now you could really get your money's worth. They were few and far between when they first started; but now there is one in practically every town. The problem with this is, once you see the food, you start eating the food. Even the best intentions are led astray when the lure of a table full of desserts is at the end of the buffet. Even if you think you don't eat much, it's not the volume that matters, it's the absorbed calories. If the restaurant doesn't list the calories or have them available, it's because the food isn't low in calories! If you eat something other than raw fruits and vegetables, the calories are approximately 100 per ounce. That means the average plate full is over 1,200 calories!

The main problem with food technology is that the ill effects linger in our body for a lifetime if you don't detoxify. This will impede weight loss and increase hunger because the body processes your nutrients inefficiently. The pesticides, herbicides, chemical fertilizers, and preservatives build up in the liver. This in turn results in increased hunger because the liver is not able to process the vitamins and minerals that you consume as efficiently as it should be. The best thing a dieter can do to deter hunger is to eat natural and organic food. It's important that you stave off the lure of the food giants, which will eventually make you giant if you're not a clever shopper.

13. PSEUDO FOOD

If I had to trace the history of the first pseudo food, I would say it all started with "If you think it's butter, it's not." This chapter will point out several dietary pitfalls that occur when you consume pseudo food.

The first problem is *over-consumption*. Suppose you decide you're going to make a diet macaroni and cheese casserole, so you assemble the recipe and grate some fat-free cheese on the top and bake it. (I always made a joke at diet meetings about the pseudo cheese that looks so much like its plastic wrapping that I don't know which one is which, let alone if the cheese inside tastes any better than the plastic.) You go to serve dinner and much to your surprise, the cheese has dried up and turned a charcoal color! You then start to eat, and the first thing that comes to mind is, *my cheese has no taste!* You continue to eat the recipe because you're waiting for the satisfaction to kick in, but it doesn't happen. Then before you know it, you've eaten twice as much as you normally would, just to comfort yourself. Besides, it's lower in calories, so why not have another portion?

Remember, the reason you purchased the fat-free cheese in the first place was to reduce your calories, but that didn't happen because you ended up eating more of the pseudo cheese than if it were real gourmet cheddar cheese. When food is reduced in anything, we tend to overeat it because we've made a sacrifice, and after all it's diet food, so why not have more?

SUGAR FREE

The food industry has reinvented food every time a dietary trend brings about consumer demand. The first of the major pseudo foods was the sugar-free group meant for diabetics. When saccharin was invented, it seemed like a logical solution to the diabetic dilemma. Now they could have their cake and eat it too. It seemed too good to be true, because it was. When we alter food from its naturally occurring state, there will always be side effects to our health.

The products made the food producers rich, yet the rates of obesity and diabetes were still on the rise. This is because the primary cause of the disease was not being addressed. The average diabetic ate more of the sugar-free product than they normally would consume, because it didn't contain sugar. This resulted in weight gain and future health problems. That trend was taking them in the wrong direction. (In contrast, when many of the type II diabetics lost weight, they no longer had the disease.)

That was only the beginning of the numerous maladies related to consuming sugar-free products. They later put warnings on the label that saccharin could cause cancer, and the consumers still purchased the products! The public was coerced by ingenious advertising that these products would replace their traditional sweets and that they could eat the food in unlimited amounts. The sugar-free pseudo food did more harm than anyone ever imagined! It's important to realize that you cannot just eat the whole package or container of a food just because the word "low" or "free" is in its name.

LOW FAT

The next dietary craze was the low-fat era. The industry was reaming out new low-fat items on a daily basis. They seemed to have accomplished the impossible. They were producing food that was once considered taboo while dieting, and now it was all right to eat all the wrong foods without guilt. When it first happened, I remember telling one of my clients that it's inherently unbelievable. The client told me she was serving a fat-free ham for Easter, and I sat back in my chair and laughed, because all I wanted to know is where did they find the fat-free pig in order to make the ham!

It's a fact that all animals are fattened up before their slaughter, because meat is sold by the pound. The more it weighs, the more it pays! In the case of the pig, it's even more outlandish because they contain so much body fat that on a winter day, a pig can appear frozen to a farmer because their fat hardens, and they feel stiff!

Dieters were ecstatic when they thought they could have cakes, cookies, candy, and desserts without any fat! The problem once again was the mere fact the food was not calorie free! The sales of the fat-free food were soaring and so was the weight of the consumers that purchased these products.

LOW CARB

The next pseudo food craze was the low-carb category. This was a whole new breed of food. Once again, it seemed like scientists had done the impossible. A consumer could purchase bread that wasn't bread and a multitude of different cakes, cookies, candies, desserts, and assorted snack items. The driving force behind these products was of course profit, and lots of it! The new low-carb food was selling for $32 per pound! That's more expensive than lobster, Alaskan king crab, and filet mignon. There were new companies investing in this cash cow on a daily basis. The only one that wasn't making out was the consumer. They were paying twice the amount of money for half the quality!

The first problem with this low-carb pseudo food was the label. They had more discrepancies than the Watergate tapes! The main selling point was that the food was supposed to be low carb. This industry created the most controversial label known to mankind. It didn't take long for the FDA to catch up with them, and the aftermath brought the low-carb fad to a severe halt in sales and profits! The reason the FDA came into the picture in the first place was that the labels made no sense at all. The nutrition facts box would state that the products contained 30 grams of carbs, yet the front of the label would claim that the food only contained 2 grams of carbs. The FDA and the consumers had one huge question to ask of the unscrupulous low-carb food companies: where did the other 28 grams of carbs go? The producers basically were caught lying on their labels, so they quickly devised a plan in order to justify their claims. This was just another ploy by the low-carb industry to appease the FDA and continue to deceive the public.

The main reason for the downfall of the low-carb pseudo food was the mere fact that eating this type of product didn't result in weight loss. There has never been a shred of scientific evidence that indicates a stable blood sugar level causes weight loss. In fact, there are millions of diabetics who are still overweight even after decades of monitoring and maintaining their blood sugar levels!

When low-carb food sales were soaring, so too were the rates of obesity in the United States. The back draft of this pseudo food fad was enormous. It left Americans with the highest rates of obesity in history! The underlying factor was once again the calories. The low-carb food was higher in calories than the real food it replaced. Therefore the more you ate of the low-carb food, the more weight you gained. The labels were designed to distract you from the most important number on the label: the calories. It doesn't matter how low in carbs a food is because your body only counts net calories when it comes to weight loss. It is important that you don't let yourself get caught up in the hype and advertising of pseudo food. This only misleads you and prolongs the inevitable, which in this case is to face the fact that net calories are the number you need to keep track of in order to lose weight!

It sounds like the low-carb scam is over, but "let the buyer beware" because these companies will not back down. They have a new concept in mind to stimulate their sales. They're going to take their low-carb products that didn't sell and put on a new label. The latest label will give the product a whole new look and shall bear the name *low G.I.* food. This new breed of food is the latest brainchild of the low-carb industry. They realize that their original endeavor was a washout and it's time to get back to the drawing board to make more money. In most cases, the label will be changed, but the product inside will remain the same. It's another lure to catch the innocent dieter looking to feed upon something that doesn't result in weight loss. The major stumbling block for this category of food is the controversy surrounding the method that actually determines the G.I. of each individual product.

The Glycemic Index is a measurement of the rate that a food enters the blood stream and its effect on blood glucose levels. The problem here is that the so-called low G.I. products usually contain several types of sugars. Some of these sugars enter the bloodstream much quicker than others, so the combining of several ingredients into one finished product changes the overall G.I. Therefore some companies list an average G.I. even though their products contain sugar, which definitely raises the blood glucose immediately.

The issue here is that the precise effect on your blood sugar is not the direct result of the product's G.I. ranking. Don't let the food giants' ingenious marketing schemes determine what you purchase and consume while dieting. There is no valid scientific evidence that this food will ever result in weight loss! You could eat low G.I. food all day and actually end up gaining weight because you ignored the most important number on the label: the calories!

ARTIFICIAL FLAVORS

The reason you crave high-calorie processed food is not all in your stomach or in your mind. There are things going on behind the scenes of the food industry that they'd rather not divulge to the average consumer. As a chemical engineer, I am aware of the fact that over 70 percent of your grocery store food is made with ingredients from a very sophisticated laboratory. When a product states that it contains artificial flavors, there can be hundreds of them in your food. Not only can artificial flavors increase your risk of cancer, but they can stimulate sensory neurons in the brain that cause you to crave the substance, no matter how much you eat of it. Therefore, even if you're full, your brain keeps telling you to eat it. Most food scientists agree that if these artificial flavors were invented today, they would have to be chemically classified as drugs! Now you won't have to wonder why one potato chip or cookie isn't enough. Isn't it about time that dieters stop letting the food giants take advantage of us? Our hard-earned money is being spent on food that contains little or no nutritional value and only leaves us with a burning desire to eat more! *This is a travesty to the American public.*

THE COLOR OF FOOD

What exactly determines the choices we make when we decide to eat one food over another? Everyone has a favorite color of M&M's, Lifesavers, jellybeans, and hard candy, just to name a few examples of foods that are selected for consumption by color. The food industry knows that eye appeal is a primary factor in purchases, and they use the lure of color to increase their sales.

The first company that artificially dyed their pistachios red made a startling deduction. The public was purchasing more of the brightly-colored nuts versus the cream-colored competition. It's a scientific fact that the human eye is drawn to a bright, vibrant color when compared to light and gentle colors. The food giants were at it again. They had devised a plan to save them money and stimulate purchases, all in one fell swoop! Their food scientists were inventing artificial colors in order to spruce up their products and attract consumers to their goods. The first problem resulting from this process was the fact that artificial food coloring can increase your chances of diseases such as cancer!

The second issue is directly related to over-consumption. Many foods that contain artificial color generally contain artificial flavor as well. These companies added cheaper, inferior ingredients to increase their profit margin. The state of your health or well-being never entered into the picture. When you're dieting, it's paramount to your success that you enjoy the food that you eat. If you buy an item that's artificially colored, you're going to experience a mental letdown, so to speak, because it's pseudo food. The product will look better than it tastes. The brain expects a certain flavor when you consume food. If, for instance, you buy an artificially colored and flavored red raspberry ice cream, you really haven't consumed what you were looking for in the first place, which was the flavor of a red raspberry. You feel compelled to eat more, hoping to eventually reach the point of satisfaction. When my dieters eat these types of pseudo food, they always comment that now they're in search of the real thing.

The perfect example came from a childhood story of one of my diet clients named Florence. Her family owned 17 acres of land in the country, and one of these acres was covered with wild blueberry bushes. As a child, she enjoyed berries on her morning cereal and in other numerous recipes like muffins and pies and as a delicious ice cream topping. The one thing Florence would not purchase when she was shopping was foods that contain artificial blueberry coloring and flavoring. She once tried a breakfast cereal with pseudo blueberry flavoring and threw away the remainder of the box. Florence stated that it left her wanting more!

ZERO TRANS FAT

The latest trend in the pseudo food category is *the zero trans fat* label. This is a particularly alarming new development in food marketing. The ploy here is when your brain sees the number zero, you give your body the liberty of having unlimited or increased portions of the food. It gives the connotation that you need not worry because there are zero grams of that nasty fat that clogs your arteries and causes heart disease. It gives the food an unwritten seal of approval because zero just simply can't add up to anything. This is just a label trick that is specifically intended to make their product appear to be healthy and useful in promoting weight loss.

Now let's turn the product around and read the nutrition "facts" box. There seems to be a significant discrepancy when you get down to the real truth regarding the calories and total fat content of this food product that claims zero trans fat. I'm going to use a bag of potato chips as my example because everyone knows they're not considered a diet food. The front of the label has a big "0" grams of trans fat written in bold across the bag. Then we turn it around only to discover it contains 150 calories per ounce and 10 grams of fat per ounce! The 8-ounce bag really adds up to 80 grams of fat, which is much larger than zero.

The major problem with pseudo food is the sheer fact that it's not designed specifically for weight loss. It is produced in order to make money. Here's a perfect example of this type of moneymaking scheme gone astray. The Hain Celestial Group decided to cancel 500 products, which were worth $15 million in annual sales. They decided that due to the decline in sales of low-carb products, producing the food wasn't worth their while. As a consumer, you must keep in mind that food is produced in order to yield profits and not to help you lose weight. The other obvious example is the Atkins' Nutritionals Inc. Their company has decided to discontinue many of their low-carb products also.

There are thousands of pseudo diet products on the market. The only way to discern one product from the other is to look at the total caloric content of the food you purchase. The mere fact that billions of dollars are spent on so-called diet food and yet our country's rates of obesity are at an all-time high speaks volumes for itself. Let's make sure that "We won't get fooled again!" as long as we are armed with truthful, logical information and adhere to the laws of science. The only real diet products are the foods that are low in net calories; because that's the number you're counting. The other so-called facts and figures just distract you from the pertinent information. So, forget the pseudo food and eat the real thing!

14. IT'S ONLY BABY FAT!

It's an American epidemic, yet no one wants to address the real issue, which is that children are consuming too many net calories. There are numerous publications and reports detailing how horrific the figures have become. The media has repeatedly announced that American children are eating more processed fast foods and exercising less. The news articles portray the parents as innocent bystanders who have no control whatsoever over their children's food choices. Another trend is to blame one specific type of food or beverage for the weight gain. There are numerous articles pointing the finger at soda and sugar consumption, while others implicate the increased intake of fast food as the culprit. The mistake here is to focus only on the causes of obesity without offering a solution to the problem. My sole purpose is to teach parents and their children how to lose weight and develop habits that result in a life that is free from obesity!

There are also the proponents who advocate healthful substitutions in order to ward off childhood obesity. They consistently attack soda and sugar-sweetened beverages as one of the largest contributors of excessive weight gain. Their solution is to drink fruit juice because it's supposedly better for your children. I have a sneaky suspicion that the marketing is designed and supported by the owner of a large juice company in order to boost their sales. If you look at the substitution theory from a mathematical standpoint, it doesn't result in weight loss. If your child was drinking soda at 150 calories per 12-ounces, and you give him fruit juice instead, which is 180 calories per 12-ounce serving, you're adding 30 more calories.

The other common food exchange is to feed your child low-fat cookies or snacks instead of the regular high-fat version. The problem here is, once again, the calories are consumed. This type of food often has 125 calories per ounce instead of the usual 150 calories per ounce. The main concern is that parents let their children eat more of it. "Why not let Junior eat the whole bag of those chips? They're low fat, so why can't he have more of them?" The simple fact is that these types of foods are still high in calories and low in nutrition. Even if your child eats only a slightly larger amount of the reduced-fat chips, he or she could actually be getting more calories!

I've had plenty of clients complain about eating junk food because they purchased it for their children. Why would you buy junk food for your children? Do you want them to become my diet clients in the future? I then ask them what they do with junk in their garage or attic when they're cleaning, and they reply, "I throw it out." Then I reply, "Then throw out your junk food!" There is no excuse for feeding your child food that is considered high-calorie junk, and if you don't feed it to them in the first place, they'll never develop a yearning for this useless food.

Some parents claim it's not their fault that their children want fast food. They blame TV's bombardment of commercials, which lure their children into wanting unhealthy food. It's time to take responsibility and turn this all around and become the proud parents of slim and trim children. The way to do this is simple when you follow my directions. You are the parents, and it's time to use your authority to help your children succeed at weight loss.

FROM THE BEGINNING

It starts from the moment your precious little bundle of joy arrives home from the hospital. The relatives "goo" and "gaa" and utter strange noises over your child in an effort to render a smile from your bambino. They pinch little Junior's cheeks and comment about how cute and plump your newborn is. It's acceptable to have a chubby child because everyone tells the parents not to worry: "It's only baby fat." Then, as your toddler begins to grow up, no one wants to be the one to deny a child food. How dare they! If the baby wants to eat the food, then give the little one exactly what he desires. If the youngster starts to develop rolls of fat, your relatives and friends tell you that Junior will "grow out" of this stage, and the baby fat will just disappear while growing up. The fact that our society accepts obesity in children as a passing phase is part of the problem of the increasing rate of childhood obesity. If you allow your child to consume anything they want, then when will the eating frenzy stop? The mere act of accepting your child's obesity sends a deeper message. It tells your child that the behavior is satisfactory and can be continued. It's your responsibility to admit that baby fat turns into adolescent fat and eventually produces an obese adult.

HOW OBESITY REALLY FEELS

The family may be willing to overlook their child's weight problem, but the rest of the world is not as kind. As a parent, you must understand that growing up as an overweight child is brutal. Their schoolmates consistently ridicule and harass them on a daily basis. I have had some young clients who dreaded the social abuse so much that they tried to quit school all together. If you could hear the cruel and degrading statements that were uttered by your child's classmates, it would bring tears to your eyes. The time has come to admit to yourself as a parent that having an overweight child is not just something they will grow out of. If you keep making excuses for your child's obesity, eventually your child will adopt those reasons for themselves and use them to remain overweight for the rest of their lives. I know I sound a bit extreme, but I speak from experience, and I don't want other children to have to endure the social punishment my family had to deal with on a daily basis.

It's important that you discuss the peer pressure that ensues with your child and develop an honest rapport with them in regard to their weight. If you just ignore the fact that they need to lose weight because you're afraid it will hurt your child's feelings, then you're only making matters worse. Childhood is a time to be carefree and happy, not depressed and obese! Let's face it, growing up and maturing into a successful adult is difficult enough as it is, so why make your child go through it overweight?

Let me give you an example of the social impact of obesity from a personal perspective. It's one of the first motivations that prompted me to become a family diet coach. It all started when my sister Sheila was born with a physical deformity. She had two club feet, and it was a true blessing that her pediatrician also had the same physical malady; he was determined to solve the problem so that others would not have to walk with permanent braces as he himself had to endure. Sheila came home in a partial body cast with hope that when it was removed she would be able to walk with the aid of corrective shoes. The weeks passed, and soon the day arrived to remove her cast. Our family was elated with the news that her surgery was successful and she was expected to have use of both her feet. It took a huge burden off our family, and the events that took place thereafter were a result of using food to show their love and gratitude for their child. My family was so ecstatic about my sister's anticipated recovery that they wanted to express their love, and the best way they knew how was by pleasing her with food.

As the years passed by, she regained full use of both her feet. This was a weight off everyone's shoulders but hers. The burden of the physical disability was removed and another was put into place; that was the affliction of obesity. The family responded by overlooking the issue of her weight problem. When the other children would ridicule her, my grandfather decided to console her by giving her the nickname "Miss America." The day finally came for her to go to school. Sheila looked forward to this day for years because she was the youngest sibling, and she wanted to follow in her older brother and sister's footsteps.

It really took her by surprise when her classmates began calling her rude and degrading names. Sheila would come home from school and cry, which didn't encourage her to want to go back the next day. She constantly tried to avoid the peer pressure of school by not attending. The repercussion was poor grades due to lack of participation. The other area of her education that she evaded was gym class. The school we went to required all the students to wear the same outfit for physical education class. The attire was a polyester one-piece suit that had built-in shorts and top, made of a tight-fitting fabric. This was a huge deterrent for overweight students because they felt so self-conscious in this type of clothing. It resulted in my sister failing her gym class because she was ashamed of the way she looked in her gym clothes.

It was time to take action and do something about her situation before it destroyed her chances to receive a good education. My family was used to making excuses for her behavior, and they tried to make her feel better by feeding her whatever she wanted. I decided to represent my sister by pleading her case to the family. I explained that the problem was her weight, and that giving her more food only made matters worse. My family told me she would grow out of this stage and it wouldn't be nice to deny her the pleasures of her favorite foods. They didn't understand because they weren't the ones who dreaded getting on the school bus for fear of being treated as an outcast and misfit.

I decided that I would use my influence as the older sister and designated family babysitter to encourage Sheila to start losing weight. I knew that if I was going to go solo in my endeavor, there would be several obstacles to overcome. The first of these hurdles was to explain to Sheila that I was on her side, so that I wouldn't trigger a defense mechanism when I mentioned that I wanted to help her lose weight. It's common in cases of childhood obesity for the child to become so self-conscious that just the suggestion of dieting leads to rebellion or withdrawal. The most logical way to deal with this situation is to institute the diet buddy system. This is discussed in detail in the section of this book called "Diet Buddies, Foes and Traitors." When you incorporate the buddy system, it doesn't create the superiority syndrome; instead, it provides level ground on which to make a fresh start. When you show a child that you are willing to diet with them, it gives them newfound hope and encouragement. This also eliminates the feelings of isolation and embarrassment, which can result when your child diets solo. Children tend to emulate their older siblings and parents, which represents a golden opportunity when it comes to dieting. This type of plan will benefit not only the child, but the buddy dieter as well. Like the old adage states, "If they can do it, I can do it too!"

I've been the designated dieter in my family ever since I can remember, but I have no regrets. As a result, I can now help millions of others lose weight because of my many years of dieting experience. I decided to use myself as the token dieter in order to help my sister lose weight. The response was overwhelming because it encouraged other overweight family members to start dieting. I was able to help my aunts and cousins lose weight, and they are thankful for my dieting advice, which they still remember me for to the present day.

Now it's time to get down to business and put your child on a weight-reduction program. If you are overweight, I suggest that you start the diet with your child and become diet buddies. It's difficult to instruct a family member to do something you haven't even accomplished yourself. You need to lead by example, not by scolding, yelling, or ridiculing. The first thing you need to do is start a daily diet diary. If your child is too young to write it down by himself, then you do it for him. If your youngster can add and print, then let him do it himself. It's a habit that will teach him how to stay thin for the rest of his life! It's not as difficult as it sounds because most children inherently like to keep a private journal. I remember when my mom bought me my first diary, and I couldn't wait to write in my daily thoughts and goals. Then I would lock it up and put it in a safe place, because it contained my innermost secrets and reflections of my daily life. The best way to know how many calories your child needs in order to lose weight is to monitor his calories prior to dieting. If your child was consuming 5,000 calories per day, and you reduce his calories to 4,000 calories per day, he will lose approximately 2 pounds per week (depending on his level of physical activity). It's important that you know your child's starting weight and measurements, so it's time to get out the weight and measurement chart provided in the Getting Started chapter and weigh him or her in!

It's of the utmost importance that you introduce your child to dieting on a positive note. You're going to be your child's diet coach, which means that you are there to train and motivate. The first thing you must do is sit down with your child and fill out a complete list of the foods your child is willing to eat. Next, instruct your child to write down their five favorite breakfasts, lunches, dinners, and snacks. This is to determine the immediate changes that can be achieved on a daily basis. It also gives your child a glimpse of what he or she was eating and how this food led to weight gain. Now it's time to add up the calories of your child's favorite meals and detect the foods that are the highest contributors to their total daily caloric intake. You can determine this by looking at the nutrition facts on the food labels.

Now separate the high-calorie foods from the low-calorie products. If an item has 100 calories or more per ounce, it's considered calorically dense and not suitable to eat while dieting. It's important to differentiate between eligible and ineligible diet food. This determines which foods your child can consume a higher volume of without going over their daily caloric limit. It's essential for your child to feel full while dieting in order to keep them on the program.

As you review their top five lists, discern the calories of each entry. If you discover there aren't many low-calorie items on the list, then half the battle is won. Once you know what causes a problem, you can take logical steps toward a solution. You should inspect the list and mark any fruits and vegetables with an asterisk (*). If you don't see any of these foods, then it's time to introduce them into your child's diet. This is accomplished by combining them with foods that they already enjoy. As a parent, you must remember that your child can only develop a taste for the foods that you feed them. For instance, if you never fed your child broccoli, how can they grow to love it?

It's important to remember that eating habits are a learned behavior. This means that you have a golden opportunity, because as a parent you are the teacher. The golden rule in dieting is: be responsible for the calories you consume. If you let your child think that eating everything and anything in sight is acceptable, then that's just what they'll do.

THE PSYCHOLOGY OF FOOD

Putting your child on a diet involves a little psychology. As a parent, you feel an emotional impact when limiting what your child eats. After all, who wants to be the one who has to take food away from a child? What kind of parent doesn't let their youngster have dessert? I'm not talking about limiting the good kind of eating, only the abusive kind. For example, it's time for a new mindset when it comes to using food as an instrument of control. What I mean is that junk food is the traditional reward designed to motivate your child to eat a certain food, perform a duty, or act in a particular manner. Here are a few common ways that parents use food to control their children's conduct:

1. *Parents offer bad food as a reward for eating good food.* "If you eat your vegetables, you can have some delicious cake for dessert."

2. *Fattening food is the reward for a chore or other task.* "If you do your home-work and clean your room, we can go out to eat this evening." This starts a pattern of thought and behavior that can carry on to adulthood if it's not changed earlier in life. How many times have you found yourself ordering take-out food because you've finished a project at work and felt that you deserved your just reward?

3. *A bribe is given to the child for being "good."* A perfect example is a trip to the grocery store. I've heard plenty of parents tell their children that if they behave during the shopping trip, they will buy them a candy bar when they arrive at the checkout aisle. Why do you think they keep the candy there in the first place? If the only reason a child listens to your requests is to receive a treat, then when will they grow up and act in a socially acceptable manner without food compensation?

The problem with using food to control your child's behavior is that it estab-lishes a long-term relationship with food that leads to long-term obesity. The child no longer looks at food as nourishment but instead as a reward. It's a fact that humans look upon food as a form of entertainment and pleasure. In the right context and format, there's nothing wrong with this concept unless we take it to the extreme and allow it to cause obesity. There's a fine line between thinness and obesity, and you can establish the boundaries at childhood instead of waiting until your offspring are grown and have to break old habits that took 30–40 years to develop!

There are obvious reasons why children like or dislike certain foods. The foremost of these is based on their parents' and grandparents' preferences. It's a fact that tradition and family heritage play an important role in the food choices we make for our children. You don't see parents preparing foods they dislike (or choose not to eat) for their offspring. The food choices we make are often a result of generations of family favorites and secret recipes prepared by Grandma and passed down to Mom. I've asked plenty of diet clients why they prefer one food over another, and they actually don't have a definite answer. The most com-mon response is that they've been preparing food that way ever since childhood, and they kind of grew into liking it because they ate it on a regular basis. The point is that, as parents, you're in the driver's seat. What you feed your children as youngsters will determine their food selections when they become adults. It's a golden opportunity to establish slim eating habits that will last your children an entire lifetime. It's up to you to decide what your children eat. Don't let your family, friends, or the media manipulate your innocent youngsters with food.

The first diet lesson for your children to learn is that food does not equal love. I know this sounds a bit harsh at first, but the sooner they understand the simple fact that food equals calories, the quicker they'll understand weight loss. Let's take a closer look at the two psychological equations and their influence on your child's eating habits!

Old Equation: Food = Love

New Equation: Food = Calories

Let me first explain that I am fully aware that food equals much more than just calories, but our perception of its meaning determines our eating habits. I know that loving your child with food is fulfilling and provides an instant response. The perfect example is going to your grandmother's house for Sunday dinner. You and your family arrive and find Grandma in the kitchen diligently preparing your favorite cuisine. Then Grandma tells her grandchildren that there's a special treat that she's prepared for dessert. As she pulls the freshly baked cake out of the oven, the youngsters respond with smiles that look like a toothpaste commercial and eyes that would light up the night sky like a full moon. Now who wants to be the one to tell your overweight child that she's not entitled to a piece of Grandma's homemade cake? How dare you deny her the happiness that she derives from eating food that was prepared in order to please her? When loved ones prepare food to make us happy, it also gives them pleasure. They are instantly rewarded with compliments and often with hugs and kisses as well. The person who loves you and your children with food becomes an instant family hero, so to speak. They are loved and appreciated for their efforts on a regular basis. It's a temptation that's too "full-filling" to pass up. After all, aren't grandparents supposed to spoil their grandchildren?

The problem with this type of behavior is that it passes on from one generation to the next. The family favorites that Grandma prepared are then cooked by their children when they become old enough to prepare food for their families. Then you have to ask yourself one question. When will it end? Specifically, who will be the one to break out of the chains of obesity that have held your family hostage for generations? When family members prepare high-calorie food for their overweight loved ones, it sends a message to the child that basically says, "Hey, I approve. Go right ahead and eat whatever you want no matter what the consequences are!"

If your child is to have dietary success, here's an important question to answer: Is the family member that prepares the "forbidden" food overweight?

If you answered "yes" to this question, then you must recognize that the over-weight relative is purposely and willingly preparing high-calorie food that will cause weight gain for their children and grandchildren, which means they themselves are not in the mode of dieting. This is a potentially volatile situation for the dieting child.

Here are two ways to avoid the pitfalls of overeating food for the sake of love:

1. *Be honest with the people who love your family with food.* If you tell your friends and relatives in advance that your child is dieting and that it would not be proper to lure them into cheating by preparing their favorite high-calorie foods, they should be happy to oblige. If they decide that they prefer not to eliminate their dessert or snacks, then offer to bring a lower calorie replacement product. There are plenty of reduced-calorie foods on the market that taste so close to the real thing that no one will notice the difference. In either case, it's always beneficial to a dieter to plan in advance for any event that involves eating. This is important because you don't need to put your child in a situation where they feel pressured or obligated to eat a particular food because it is there.

2. *Substitute a non-food gift* to show love and appreciation to your children. If you provide a token of love in the form of a present, it lasts a lifetime instead of only a few minutes. The problem with using food as affection is that the aftermath also lasts a lifetime in the form of weight gain and eventually obesity. It only takes about 10 minutes to eat a piece of cake or pie, and all of a sudden, you've consumed 600 calories!

It's important to remember that your child's metabolism is at an all-time high and will decrease as he or she grows older. This means that it's crucial to your child's future eating habits and weight control to teach them how to reduce their calories and develop thin eating behavior. The decision to consume a low-calorie food or a high-calorie food is what determines your body weight. If your child doesn't know the difference between high- and low-calorie food, how can you expect them to make a logical selection when they decide what to eat each day? When your child is armed with appropriate knowledge, they have an opportunity to determine their "weight loss destiny."

If your child is taught how to lose weight without decreasing the volume of food they consume, then the chances for successful and permanent weight loss are tremendous. The logical starting point is to determine the foods and beverages that contribute the most calories toward their daily intake.

HIGH-CALORIE PITFALLS

Children consume plenty of *useless calories in the form of liquids*. It's mind boggling to take a gander at the beverage aisle of the grocery store. There is everything from energy drinks to functional refreshments in every flavor imaginable. The industry uses sports heroes and movie stars to advertise these products in hopes of luring our children into drinking their beverage. They are often flavored with artificial ingredients, which in turn cause the brain to crave the product even more. It's such a profitable segment of big business that some athletes make more money from doing soda commercials than they do from their sports salary. If your child is overweight, there is no reason to have him or her consume liquid calories. The best choice is pure water or a reduced-calorie beverage. The calories they consume should be in the form of food, not liquids.

Another big culprit that contributes to childhood obesity is the school lunch. I have had plenty of schoolteachers and educational staff members that gain weight as a result of eating the traditional school lunch. The proof lies in the fact that when they bring their own food to eat instead of the school's lunch, they lose weight! The first step is to have your school give you a copy of the lunch menu. Then ask the school to provide you with the calories of the meals that they're serving your child.

You probably won't get very far with that question, because the average school system doesn't even know how many calories they're feeding their students. If we don't know the facts and figures, then how can we make the right choices? The ball is in your court now, because you as a parent must decide what to feed your child for lunch. It's a fact that every child is served the same portion size in the school cafeteria whether they are normal weight or overweight. This makes no logical sense at all. The overweight child needs to reduce their calorie intake, which means the portions of high-calorie foods must be reduced. Yet, at the same time, they can increase the serving size of the low-calorie foods so that your child's lunch will be the same volume as the other students' meals.

The main problem with the current school lunch program is that the type of food being served does not promote good eating habits. The current array of cuisine reads like the menu at a typical fast-food restaurant. The fare offered consists of hamburgers, hot dogs, tacos, deep-fried chicken, mozzarella sticks, french fries, and pizza. These are obviously not the types of food that promote a healthy lifestyle. Your child can't eat these foods on a daily basis and expect to grow up liking fruits and vegetables. It's important to establish a taste for low-calorie foods in childhood, because eating habits tend to last a lifetime.

The secondary drawback is that the foods served contain little or no nutritional value. In the case of most public school systems, it's a fact that all the grains served are derived from white processed flour. The hot dog rolls, hamburger rolls, bread, and pasta are all white. The protein sources are mainly comprised of processed meats like hamburger, hotdogs, and luncheon meat. The fats are from animal sources. There is not one item on the typical school lunch program that provides your child with the essential omega-3 fats!

The problem that arises from eating food that's basically devoid of vitamins and minerals is hunger. When a student eats a lunch that deprives the body of nutrients, it's common sense that the youngster will still feel hungry when they're finished eating, because their body requires nutrients in order to grow both physically and mentally. If they're going to consume the current school lunches, then their diet should be supplemented with my natural multi-vitamin.

Let me give you a perfect example of an ordinary school lunch that's insufficient for the nutritional needs of a maturing child. The menu item is a grilled cheese sandwich with chocolate milk, french fries, peas and carrots, and a cutie pie. Now let's analyze this meal for its calorie content as well as its nutritional value. The foremost number to calculate is the total caloric content of the lunch, which is listed below. This particular meal uses four slices of bread because New York State requires at least 3 ounces of protein for each lunch that is served, regardless of the age or weight of the student. The school cook therefore decides that putting 3 ounces of cheese on one sandwich is too difficult to fit, so she uses four slices of bread so that the sandwiches aren't overflowing with melted cheese.

SCHOOL LUNCH

Grilled Cheese Sandwich:	Calories	Fat
4 slices of white bread	280	2
4 oz. American cheese	400	20
1 Tbsp. margarine	100	11
1 serving french fries	150	10
Deep fried in oil	120	14
1 serving peas & carrots	100	1
1 Tbsp. margarine	100	8
1 cutie pie	400	20
1 pint chocolate milk	340	18
	1,990 calories	104 grams of fat

The point of the example is that our children are consuming far too many calories for lunch. It's common knowledge among parents and teachers that the school lunch is designed to feed the masses for the least amount of money and yet appease the public by appearing to adhere to our children's nutritional requirements.

When you take a deeper look at what we're really feeding our children, it makes logical sense that obesity is on the rise. The amount of fat in one school lunch is more than a child should consume for the entire day! The best way to help your child lose weight is to monitor their total daily caloric intake. This means that lunch shouldn't contribute the largest amount of calories to their daily total. Your child needs to save the majority of their calories for dinner (and snack if they so desire).

There are some schools that offer a salad bar for their pupils as an alternative to their traditional fare. This appears to offer a solution for overweight students, yet there are hidden calories that will add up quickly if your child is not savvy to the pitfalls of an all-you-can-eat salad bar. The first caloric culprit is the regular salad dressing, as we have discussed. The second snare for the dieter is the unlimited portions of cheese, cottage cheese, and mayonnaise-laden items such as potato salad and pasta salad. These items are often too tempting to pass up, but they put your caloric count above the acceptable limit for lunch.

Let's take a look at how an innocent salad becomes a dieter's scorn.

SALAD BAR LUNCH

	Calories	Fat
1 C. lettuce	5	0
4 cucumber slices	4	0
2 tomato wedges	2	0
4 Tbsp. regular salad dressing	380	40
4 oz. cheese	400	28
1 C. macaroni salad	615	27
1 C. potato salad	358	26
	1,764	121

When you take the time to analyze this lunch option, it's not a worthy diet meal unless you make a couple of simple substitutions. Your child can have a large bowl of raw vegetables and use diet dressing instead of regular salad dressing. If your child still requires more sustenance, then you can pack them a low-calorie sandwich to go along with the salad for a filling and nutritious lunch.

The standard school lunch presents many obstacles for the overweight student. They are so low in volume that plenty of students have told me they need to order two lunches in order to feel satisfied. It's also common practice for students to omit the fruits and vegetables altogether and eat the main entrée and the dessert instead. The temptation for an overweight adolescent to overeat is overwhelming in this social situation. It's required by law for students to attend the school lunch break. Then the children must stand in line and make a quick dietary decision so that they don't hold up the lunch line. If they inquire about the ingredients or ask for a substitution, it's noticed by their fellow students. It's not the place where kids want to attract attention by being the picky eater.

I'll give you an example from my own school years. I'm over forty years old, and I still remember being made fun of by my peers for asking for water instead of milk at the cafeteria. I went to school in a small community called Lyncourt with only one school, which housed students from kindergarten to the ninth grade all under one roof. The institution was so small that the gymnasium was converted to the lunch area, and everyone brought their own food. I didn't like standard lunch fare, so I brought food that was out of the ordinary and as a result raised the eyebrows of my fellow students. I became so disgruntled that I eventually left my lunch in the school locker rather than become the brunt of food jokes! It got to the point where they would eventually get rancid, and the teachers were so used to my practice that when the hall smelled peculiar, they would ask me to discard my old lunches. I did this just to avoid the ridicule caused by eating differently from other students! It wasn't until I graduated from this small school that I was bussed to another town to attend high school. I had never seen the inside of a school cafeteria until I was in the tenth grade. It was a shock to the system.

The whole process was more like a chore or obligation than to satisfy nutritional needs. The school only allowed twenty minutes for lunch, and it took at least four minutes to walk to the cafeteria and four minutes to walk back to your next class. When you got to the cafeteria, the line was constant, and it took roughly five to seven minutes to purchase your food and find a seat. This left only about seven minutes to eat your entire meal! It wasn't an atmosphere conducive to sitting down and enjoying a meal. My first impression was that of a flock of sheep being herded to a field so they could graze upon the grass.

I never liked being told what to eat and when to eat, and I still don't, so this lunch ritual was not appealing to me. I then asked to take another class instead of attending the school lunch period. The school was happy to oblige, and I took

Spanish as an independent study course so that I could eat in peace or not eat if I chose to do so. Everything was fine until the board of education discovered I was breaking a state law! It's mandatory for a student to participate in school lunch in New York State. I was headed back to the cafeteria in spite of all of my efforts to avoid the place.

I've presented an extreme case in order to prove a point. I was determined not to overeat, and I did everything in my power to avoid the temptations of the school lunch. If you really want to achieve a goal, you'll do whatever it takes to accomplish your endeavor. An overweight child needs to bring their lunch to school because their program is not suitable for dieting adolescents.

TOP 12 WAYS FOR YOUR CHILD TO LOSE WEIGHT

This list is designed to help you impart small dietary changes, which will subtract calories, not volume, from your child's diet. If you alter your child's diet drastically, chances are they will feel deprived, which may lead to food binges. The purpose of dieting is weight loss, not starvation and frustration. It's important to keep your child satisfied both mentally and physically while dieting so that they will stay on the program long enough to reach their weight-loss goal.

1. REDUCE AND EVENTUALLY ELIMINATE THE CONSUMPTION OF REGULAR SODA.

It's a scientific fact that the chemicals contained in soda increase your chances of cancer and contribute to the destruction of bones and teeth. Yet, many parents give it to their children on a daily basis. The mere fact that it contains 150 calories per 12-ounce serving is reason enough to exclude it from an overweight child's diet. If your child consumes two sodas per day, that's 109,500 calories per year. If you discontinue this little habit, your child will lose up to 31 pounds by the end of the year with just this one simple dietary change! The calories contained in soda are derived from white processed sugar, which contains no valuable nutrients whatsoever. They're simply wasted calories. I don't expect your child to go cold turkey, but there is a way to make your child a low-calorie, healthy soda alternative. You simply take an organic juice and mix it with a natural seltzer. If you use 4 ounces of juice and 8 ounces of seltzer, your new version of soda will contain 80 calories instead of 150. If you're not willing to prepare a low-calorie soda for your child, then you should have them drink a diet soda, which contains zero calories!

2. STOP GIVING YOUR CHILD WHOLE MILK.

I know that for years the dairy association has told parents that milk helps your child build strong bones and teeth, but this is simply a brilliant marketing campaign. It's designed to make you feel guilty if you deny your youngster their daily dose of milk. America has the highest dairy consumption in the world, yet it also has the highest rate of osteoporosis in the world! That's because the human body is designed to absorb calcium from sources also, like leafy green vegetables. If you're concerned about your child's intake of calcium, then purchase a chewable calcium supplement from your local natural food store that is proven to be bio-available. This way your child receives their daily dose of calcium without consuming any calories. It always strikes me as odd that parents are concerned with this one mineral because of fervent advertising, but they don't seem to worry about the other vitamins and minerals their child needs on a daily basis to keep them healthy!

If your child drinks three 8-ounce glasses of whole milk per day, that equals 164,250 calories per year. If you simply eliminate this habit, your youngster will lose up to 47 pounds by the end of the year! Now take a moment to see how much you're actually serving your child, because it determines the calories saved and, in turn, the projected weight loss. Just fill a glass with the amount of milk you typically give your child. Then get a measuring cup and find out how much milk is in the glass. Each 8-ounce cup has 150 calories, so add up the calories. For instance, if you give your child 12 ounces of milk, then there are 225 calories per glass.

The point I'm making here is that liquid calories add up fast and go down fast, so they must be monitored and accounted for in your child's diet journal. If you find it rather difficult for your child to give up milk all at once, then reduce the calories of the milk by using skim milk, which has 90 calories per 8-ounce cup, instead of 150 calories. If the thought of skim milk is appalling to your child, then try to make a low-calorie chocolate milk for them in order to save calories. The regular grocery store chocolate milk contains up to 280 calories per cup. If your child drinks 2 cups per day of conventional chocolate milk, it adds up to 204,400 calories per year. The low-calorie version is made by taking 8 ounces of skim milk and 1-tablespoon plain cocoa, and sweeten it with stevia until the desired taste is achieved. This version contains only 95 calories per 8-ounce serving, versus 280 calories. If you serve your child this version twice a day instead of the high-calorie choice, your child could lose up to 39 pounds by the end of the year.

3. STOP GIVING YOUR CHILD CHOCOLATE!

I know what you're thinking already. "How will I get my child to stop eating chocolate?" Let's remember that the first priority here is weight loss, and this is accomplished by reducing your child's caloric intake. There are four reasons why you need to negate chocolate from their diet:

A. It's calorically dense. It contains 150 calories per ounce, and the calories add up much too quickly.

B. The product is devoid of nutrients. The traditional chocolate companies use hydrogenated oils and artificial flavors, both of which could be harmful to your child's health. If you look at chocolate in terms of dieting, it makes no sense at all to waste so many calories on so little volume. If your child consumes 3 ounces of chocolate daily at 150 calories per ounce, this will equal 164,250 calories in only 1 year!

C. The artificial flavors in the candy stimulate the brain to crave more and more without providing biological satisfaction.

D. It establishes a habit that will last a lifetime unless something is done while they're young.

If you've been using chocolate as a reward system, then find an alternative (preferably a non-food bonus) to give your child instead. There are plenty of low-calorie confections on the market that make suitable substitutions. You can buy chocolate-flavored hard candy, which has only 10 calories apiece or prepare a low-calorie hot chocolate beverage for your child to enjoy. There are an abundance of nonfat frozen yogurts and fat-free chocolate ice creams to choose from, but be careful not to over-compensate with substitutions, because it's your child's total daily caloric intake that determines their weight loss.

It's crucial to remember that eating patterns are established when your child is young. If you like chocolate when you're a child, chances are you'll grow to love chocolate as an adult. The sooner you accept the fact that chocolate is much too high in calories to be consumed by a dieter, the easier it becomes to eliminate it from your diet. So you have to ask yourself the pertinent question: "When will I stop eating like a child and start eating like an adult?"

It's a statistical fact that 78 percent of all American adults eat candy, and two-thirds of them consume chocolate candy. The real issue is how many of these candy consumers began the habit of eating sweets when they were children. If you want a realistic answer, just ask yourself when you started eating candy. The sooner you get your child out of the routine of eating sweets the better. A habit or behavior is easier to change when it has been practiced for 5 years versus 40 years!

It's time to sit down with your child and have a diet chat. The old adage "honesty is the best policy" applies perfectly to this situation. You should explain to them that the calories in chocolate are much too high to be consumed while dieting. Let them know that this type of food is contributing to their weight gain. The good news is that it's not much volume to subtract out of their diet. The benefits of giving up such a small portion are well worth the effort. It's important that your child is fully aware of the foods that cause them to gain weight, and chocolate is certainly one of them!

4. STOP TAKING YOUR CHILD TO FAST-FOOD RESTAURANTS!

There are many reasons why you should curtail your fast food visits, but the most obvious one is that the food is much too high in calories. The typical fast-food meal contains 1,200 calories, and over 50 percent of these calories come from fat. The food is processed, and therefore the nutrients are destroyed. If you take the time to really analyze what you're purchasing, it's not worth the money or the weight gain that results from eating at fast-food restaurants.

If you examine the calories of the traditional menu items offered at a fast-food eatery, it's simple to understand why you shouldn't be bringing your child there to eat. I've heard excuses pertaining to this issue, but it's time to move forward and establish reasons why you don't want to eat fast food. When a parent tells me that they don't have time to prepare a meal, so they conveniently pick up fast-food meals, my first response is to chuckle in order to quell my anger, because I realize this is just another excuse to consume unhealthy food.

The real issue here is that the parent has decided that they also want to eat fast food. How many parents who take their children to these types of restaurants also enjoy the food themselves? If time is really an issue, then ask yourself how long it takes to dress up the children and get them into the vehicle then drive to the fast-food place, wait in line to place your order, wait in line to receive and pay for your items, and finally drive back home. The whole process takes more time than it does to get out a pan and proceed to cook a low-calorie version of their hamburger. It's amazing that the same person who told me that they were so pressed for time will find the opportunity to watch their favorite television shows and even manage to check their e-mail and surf the Internet. Your family and children are worth the time that it takes to make them a diet meal.

Another excuse commonly used by parents is that their children are coerced by ingenious marketing schemes that lure them into these restaurants. There's no doubt in my mind that the cute little prizes and so-called collectables offered free with your children's menu items have a direct influence on the youngsters.

The simple fact is that it's just an advertisement. The sooner you teach your child that the purpose of a commercial is to convince him to purchase a product, the less likely he will be taken advantage of as an adult. The very fact that fast-food restaurants are using advertising that can change your child's mind about their food choices is reason enough not to spend your hard-earned money at places that intentionally market to innocent children. It's time for the American public to take responsibility for what their children eat. After all, they represent the next generation of our society, and we want them to be healthy and intelligent. This can't be accomplished by feeding them fast food on a consistent basis.

If you look at the repercussions that result from opening a fast-food restaurant in a country that has never had such an establishment, the evidence of its presence is obvious. The first indisputable outcome is the increase in obesity. The fast-food restaurant will super-size you when it moves into your community, if you eat there. The second back draft of fast food arriving in unchartered territory is the onset of health problems such as heart disease, high cholesterol, high blood pressure, and diabetes. The statistical facts of increased health maladies are staggering enough to keep a health- or weight-conscious individual from ever entering its doors.

Another problem associated with the consumption of fast food is the time factor. I refer to the fact that the food is soft and mushy, which involves a limited amount of chewing. This type of food is typically consumed quickly, which is usually counter-productive to dieting. If you only have a limited amount of calories that you can eat in one day, you should enjoy and savor each and every one of them. I'll give you a perfect example of how quickly calories can be consumed. A woman pulled up in her van and parked in front of my natural food store. I was curious because she didn't get out and come into the store. I took a look at what she was doing, and I noticed she was eating a Big Mac. I shouldn't say the word eating, because what it looked like she was doing was shoving it down her throat. In about a minute, the Big Mac was gone, and her hands were foraging into a bag that she had placed in her lap to get yet another Big Mac! The second one was consumed in the same manner as the first. She didn't seem to be enjoying herself at all. It was as though she were on a mission instead of having dinner. She actually reminded me of those people you see in the burger-eating contests. After her second Big Mac, she pulled out a bag of large fries and a soda. She proceeded to gobble up the fries very quickly. Her mouth was still full when she devoured the next bite. It only took her about five minutes to consume 2,000 calories! The moral of the story is that fast food is eaten much too quickly and has a high caloric density. It's important not to let your child get into the fast-food habit, because chances are it will become a permanent habit that contributes to a lifetime of obesity and health problems. Now is the time to establish low-calorie eating patterns that will give your child the opportunity to mature into a healthy adult.

5. IT'S TIME TO GIVE YOUR CHILD'S SNACK A LOW-CALORIE MAKEOVER.

It's a typical event in the everyday life of a child to have an after-school or evening snack. I'm not going to tell you to have your child go cold turkey or ask you to give him celery sticks as a snack, because it's just not a logical solution to the snack dilemma. It always amazes me when you pick up a magazine that comments on how horrible the childhood obesity epidemic is and then proceeds to tell you the answer to the problem is as simple as feeding them more fruits and vegetables and making them exercise. This looks lovely in print, but how much of their advice actually comes to fruition? It's typical of the diet industry to tell you what to do and assume you will automatically follow the instructions to a tee. The articles published on childhood obesity don't even take the time to mention the *c* word.

The major problem with the snack habit is they contain far too many calories and little or no nutritive value. If your child has the practice of eating four cookies with a glass of milk after school, this little indulgence can add up to 550 calories. If your child is used to consuming products that contain processed sugar, hydrogenated oils, and artificial colors, they tend to develop food addictions. When will your children stop eating sweet snacks? There's no better time than the present to serve them suitable diet snacks. There are plenty of low-calorie cookies on the market, which are great impersonators of their high-calorie competitors. When you do make a snack substitution, it's important to account for the total calories that your child consumes. It's common practice for rookie dieters to overeat a low-calorie food because they don't count their total caloric intake each day.

The second most commonly served snack falls into the crunchy, salty category. This is the type of snack that is commonly described by consumers as follows: "Once I have one, I'll eat the whole bag!" It's amazing that even though a person knows the impending doom of the consequences of purchasing these snack foods, they still buy them and give them to their family. There are several changes that can be made in order to decrease your child's snack calories. The first rule of thumb is to stop serving the snack directly from the bag. If, for instance, you put a bag of chips on a dining room table, you're sending out a subliminal message that states, "Go ahead and eat this because it's here for the taking, and it's all right to eat the whole bag." The new diet snack rule is to serve the snack in a small bowl. This automatically reduces the calories and establishes a serving size. Snacks like potato chips, corn chips, cheese curls, etc., contain 150 calories per ounce. This means an 8-ounce bag of conventional snacks contains 1,200 calories. The best way to encourage healthier snack habits is to practice the Party Mix Theory. The main point of this theory is to mix the calories of your high-calorie food with low-calorie products in order to lower the total caloric content of the snack. It's also mentally appealing because the dieter still gets the pleasure of eating the same volume and doesn't have to entirely eliminate her favorite munchies.

The major reason consumers can't stop eating these crunchy creations is because they may contain artificial flavors that cause the brain to crave more and more of them, similar to drugs that cause addiction. It's a wise idea to change your snacks from regular grocery store brands to an organic natural type in order to reduce the level of craving. Natural food is much more satisfying because the flavor is real. Therefore, the brain can recognize the flavor and register it in its memory as fulfilling a desire for that particular taste it was looking for in the first place. It's paramount to dieting success that the dieter doesn't feel cheated or deprived. You can't expect your child to sit and watch the rest of the family eat chips and dip while he munches on crudités. It's time to try the party mix theory, and the best snack to use is good old-fashioned popcorn. It's important that you purchase the proper type of popcorn because this product can be highly adulterated and end up containing as many calories as potato chips. The two numbers you need to pay close attention to are the calories and the total amount of servings per package.

You should calculate the total number of calories in the whole bag of popcorn so that the serving size is adjusted for that particular day's caloric limit. The next step is to prepare your party mix. The individual ingredient choices are dependent on your child's personal preference for snacks. If for instance your child will eat pretzels, then you can mix them into your popcorn for variety and to help reduce the caloric content of the snack. Listed below are several items that spruce up any bowl of popcorn and provide multiple tastes, which in turn render an increased level of satisfaction for your child's pleasure.

PARTY MIX OPTIONS

Snack	Net calories Per ounce	Snack	Net calories Per ounce
Low-calorie popcorn	25-50 per C.	Raw Nuts and Seeds	
Pretzels	100 per oz.	(Organic is best)	

Dried Fruit		Almonds	102
(Organic is best)		Brazil nuts	108
Apples	48 per oz.	Cashews	100
Apricots	46 per oz.	Filberts	105
Cranberries	59 per oz.	Macadamia nuts	102
Dates	54 per oz.	Peanuts	100
Figs	50 per oz.	Pecans	114
Mangos	59 per oz.	Pistachio nuts	96
Pineapples	60 per oz.	Pumpkin seeds	96
Raisins	58 per oz.	Soy nuts	70
Organic raw trail mix	88 per oz.	Sunflower seeds	89
		Walnuts	114

Let's examine the above list and make sure that the items you use are suitable for the party mix. The main reason that organic fruits, nuts, and seeds are chosen is that they contain more nutrients than their conventional grocery store competitors. The new snack you've prepared now provides your child with essential nutrients instead of wasted calories. In addition, the numerous chemicals used on pesticide-ridden food can destroy brain cells and may cause cancer, as well as a host of other maladies. The choice is yours as a parent. I'm just providing you with the scientific facts so that you can make a logical decision when you purchase these items.

The main detail you need to pay particularly close attention to is that the nuts and seeds should be raw. Raw food provides the human body with enzymes that help to expedite digestion. This in turn results in faster weight loss. Most raw items also contain a high-fiber content, which is advantageous to weight loss.

The party mix examples illustrate the fact that there are numerous possibilities available for low-calorie snack sensations. The main point of the party mix theory is to reduce the calories per ounce of your child's snack. This results in lowering your youngsters' total daily caloric intake.

6. REDUCE YOUR CHILD'S FAT INTAKE, ESPECIALLY THE CONSUMPTION OF BUTTER, MARGARINE, AND OIL.

It's a typical scene—breakfast time at the household of the average American family. The children are rushing to the table while Dad goes over some last-minute paperwork and Mom prepares the family breakfast as she gets ready for the office. The scent of eggs and toast is in the air as Mom places a tub of margarine on the kitchen table. The butter knife is set next to it, and each member of the family is responsible for deciding how much margarine they will use on their bread.

The first problem with this scene is that the utensil used to serve the margarine is a butter knife, which doesn't indicate any portion size. If your child doesn't know the difference between a teaspoon and a tablespoon, how can you expect them to control their portion sizes? It's time to take your measuring spoons out of the cupboard and use them to determine how much butter or margarine your child is putting on her toast. If you measure out a level teaspoon of butter and put it on toast, you'll realize that your child has probably been using closer to a tablespoon on each slice of bread, which adds up to 200 calories instead of 60 calories. If you take a closer look at how many calories the average family consumes in the form of pure fat, the figures are quite alarming. The typical family of four purchases a 18 oz. bottle of oil and a 16-ounce tub of margarine or butter per week. The oil is 4,320 calories per bottle, and the margarine or butter is 3,200 calories per tub, totaling 7,520 calories. If the family consumes the fat equally, then the two children have 25 percent each. This equates to 1,880 calories per week totaling 97,760 calories per year. This means up to 28 pounds of weight gain per child in only one year!

The central truth of the matter is that fat contains nine calories per gram. This means that the more fat a food has, the more calories it contains overall. The worst-case scenario of wasting calories occurs when a child unknowingly loads butter, margarine, or oil on a food out of sheer habit. The actual fat itself doesn't add volume or taste to the food; it just adds a tremendous amount of calories to the meal. It's a dietary shame to pour oil on an innocent salad. The best way to reduce your child's fat intake is to start with the obvious diet violations. The products that derive all of their calories from fat should be the first place to make changes. The following is a list of such items. In order to make simple dietary replacements, refer to the Calorie Saving Substitution List in this book.

Fat	Cal. per oz.	Fat	Cal. per oz.
Butter	215	Sunflower oil	240
Coconut oil	240	Margarine	204
Corn oil	240	Soft margarine	200
Cotton seed oil	240	Stick	200
Crisco oil	240	Tub	200
Olive oil	240	Corn oil margarine	200
Palm oil	240	Safflower margarine	200

Palm kernel oil	240	Soy margarine	200
Peanut oil	240	Vegetable margarine	200
Safflower oil	240	Mayonnaise	200
Sesame oil	240	Vegetable oil	240
Soybean oil	240		

The second condiment group that needs to be excluded from a dieting child's intake is regular salad dressing. The most common diet fallacy is that vinaigrettes are somehow lower in calories than traditional salad dressings. The name itself is misleading because it implies that the product is mainly comprised of vinegar, which contains a miniscule amount of calories and is usually put on the calorie-free list. If you take a look at the order of ingredients in the average vinaigrette, there's more oil than vinegar. Then take a gander at the calories, and you'll realize this is not a low-calorie condiment. The average calories of a vinaigrette are 100 per ounce. The typical child pours at least 2 ounces of dressing on their salad, which means they just put 200 calories of liquid on their food. If you purchase diet salad dressing, they will be saving at least 150 calories every time they eat a salad. Remember, the items that adorn your food should add flavor, not calories.

7. KICK THE SUGAR HABIT; YOUR CHILD IS ALREADY SWEET ENOUGH.

If you open up your kitchen cupboards right now and examine the contents, how many different items will you find that would fall into the sweets category? It's a fact that the per capita consumption of sugar in the United States is 153 pounds per year. At 1,702 calories per pound, that adds up to 260,406 calories per year, or 74 pounds of potential weight gain. When you take the time to really calculate the calories wasted on sugar, the figures are astounding.

Now let's continue with your "sweet" inspection. This lesson will provide ample evidence that desserts are much too calorically dense for your child to consume on a regular basis. First, gather all the sweet snacks in your house and put them on your table, making sure you include the frozen treats in your freezer. Next, add up the total calories, including the whole box of cookies and the entire half-gallon of ice cream. Then take the grand total and divide by the number of days it takes to consume them. For example:

Item	Calories	Servings	Total calories
Chocolate chip cookies	140	8	1,120

Sandwich cookie	130	12	1,560
Oatmeal cookie	130	10	1,300
Chocolate chip cookie dough	300	16	4,800
Vanilla & chocolate frozen bars	350	8	2,800
Chocolate bars	150	12	1,800
Chocolate cup cakes	250	12	3,000
Cinnamon Buns	510	12	6,120
Glazed donut	310	12	3,720
			26,220

A family of four with two children compiled the above list of items. The household will consume these calories within two weeks, which adds up to 26,220 calories/2 weeks, equaling 13,110 calories in one week. This converts to 13,110 calories/4 people, equaling 3,277 calories per person. Over a year, each person will consume 170,404 calories. This could lead to a weight gain of 49 pounds for each family member in only one year. This doesn't even take into account the consumption of desserts that are eaten at restaurants and parties outside of the home.

The latest trend in our culture is to celebrate children's birthdays with a gala event. The stories I hear in reference to planning birthday parties sound more like the makings of a wedding than a child's party. It's commonplace now for a family to rent out a restaurant, skating rink, or pizza parlor for their youngster's birthday. When you consider the financial and dietary ramifications, it's not a feasible plan. The primary reason that this isn't a suitable idea for an overweight child is that there are too many temptations. The typical birthday party fare is comprised of cake, ice cream, chips, pizza, and other assorted high-calorie snack foods. It's not realistic to ask your child to go to a party and refrain from eating while they watch all their friends eat whatever they desire.

There is a viable solution to the traditional birthday bash. It's time to organize a parental think tank. I'm asking you as a parent of an overweight child to meet with other parents in your social unit who also have kids who need to lose weight. The purpose of this gathering is to plan a unique new type of birthday party: a place where children can have fun without gaining weight as a result of high-calorie foods offered to them at the party.

This can be accomplished in a number of ways. The primary food that needs dietary alteration is the birthday cake. As discussed, the average piece of cake contains between 500–800 calories. This is far too many calories for an overweight child to consume in one single serving of food. There are plenty of low-calorie recipes that can be prepared in lieu of the customary birthday cake. There are fat-free brownie mixes on the market that taste so rich and creamy that even the most discerning taste buds wouldn't know that it's not the high calorie version. You can top this sweet sensation with a low-calorie ice cream or frozen yogurt for a special treat. There are plenty of delicious low-calorie snacks available to replace the conventional high-calorie chips. See the Party Mix section of this book for more scrumptious solutions.

If you plan to serve the children a meal, then have the parents each bring a low-calorie version of the customary cuisine. A perfect example is pizza because the difference in calories between a restaurant version and a homemade one is phenomenal. Once your children get a taste of a freshly baked pizza, they won't be asking you to order out, because they'll be asking to help spread the dough for the pizza instead.

8. IT'S IMPORTANT THAT YOUR CHILD ACQUIRES ANOTHER HOBBY BESIDES EATING.

The predominant portion of our entertainment in this country involves eating. There are plenty of families that celebrate the weekend by going out to dinner. It gives us a chance to reflect upon the week and enjoy some time with our loved ones. It's difficult enough for an adult to control their caloric intake while eating, so just imagine the impact it has on your child. The child's menu usually consists of hot dogs and hamburgers, which aren't a dieter's best friend by any stretch of the imagination. Remember, the habits we acquire at childhood tend to stay with us throughout our lives. Therefore, it's important to develop traditions that help us to maintain a normal body weight.

I'm not asking you to refrain from eating out altogether. Instead, I'm urging you as a parent to take them to a restaurant that offers lower-calorie food items. What do you expect your child to order when you take them to a pizza parlor? It's not logical to ask your overweight child to eat a salad with low-calorie dressing while the rest of the family munches on pepperoni pizza.

If eating is a significant pastime for your child, you need to help them procure a new hobby. One alternative is a trip to the local sports card store. This will light up any child's eyes when they see their favorite athlete's photo and stats on a baseball or football card. If you use the money you would have spent at the restaurant, then your budget stays the same. However, your child now has a permanent memory of the time you have spent money together, instead of just a crumpled bag in the garbage that housed some high-calorie food items.

It's important that you give your overweight child an opportunity to develop hobbies other than eating. When a youth begins a collection, it tends to become a project that lasts for many years. It teaches your adolescent to appreciate the value of things other than food. Their mind is occupied with thoughts of how to procure appropriate souvenirs like cards in order to complete their collection instead of what snack to munch upon next.

There are endless options available for children to collect or build things. It's always an accomplishment to finish a jigsaw puzzle, and it's an activity your children can enjoy together. It's time to have a chat with your child and ask them what craft or hobby they would like to begin doing. If they're unsure of their hidden talents, then help them unleash their creativity with a trip to a craft store or a science shop. You'll be amazed as a parent by the aptitude children have when they're given the opportunity to excel in new-found hobbies and activities other than eating!

The most obvious activity that you can encourage your overweight child to participate in is an athletic endeavor. I'm not asking you to turn Junior into an athlete, but if this is what happens as a result, then it's an additional bonus for your child. The main goal is to burn additional calories through some sort of physical activity. This not only accelerates weight loss but also boosts your child's metabolism. The other benefit of encouraging and involving your child with exercise and sports is that it teaches discipline.

There are numerous options available for increasing your child's level of physical activity. The best way to proceed is to simply ask your child what sports they're interested in joining. This gives them the ability to participate because they prefer this type of exercise, not because their parents are forcing them to do so. If you expect your child to be diligent and consistent at any type of activity, it should be something they have an interest in pursuing. If your child is unde-cided, then it's time to shop around for the suitable sport. It should be one that they will benefit from and look forward to participating in, such as group classes, private lessons, or perhaps even athletic competitions. There are many activities available for adults and children in this country, and many of the options for athletic activities are group classes that the whole family can enjoy together. When starting an exercise program, there's one simple rule that applies in order to establish a consistent routine: it has to be something your child likes.

It's not necessary to spend thousands of dollars on expensive exercise attire and equipment, which your child may only use for a short period of time before deciding that this sport isn't their forte. It's more important that you just get your child started, which establishes a routine and hopefully a habit that will last a lifetime.

There are plenty of used sports equipment stores where you can purchase sporting supplies and attire at a reduced price. If your child decides they would prefer to participate in a group sport, then find a location that allows you and your child to participate in a couple of lessons at a reduced or pro-rated price before you go ahead and sign a lengthy contract. I'll give you a perfect example of the importance of "try it before you buy it" experiences. There are plenty of children who, after they've watched the events on television, think skiing and snowboarding are exciting sports to participate in. Then the actual day comes, they go to the ski shop to purchase the equipment, and before you know it, your adolescent has chosen the best ski gloves, boots, and equipment available in the industry. As a parent, you feel obliged to encourage your child to participate in sports as a way to instill discipline and lose weight. Then before the credit card bill even arrives in the mail, your child decides that he or she doesn't really want to travel full speed down frozen tundra.

The moral of this story is not to spend thousands of dollars in order to inspire your child to participate in a sport, just proceed logically and understand that their goals and desires may change on daily basis. If you as a parent allow them an opportunity to explore the various sports and exercise options available, then they will eventually find the suitable activity and continue to participate in it on a daily basis. It's essential that you remember that the goal is to provide your child with the proper tools of the trade in order to achieve permanent weight loss, and exercise is one of these tools that allows you a dietary edge.

9. DECREASE YOUR CHILD'S CONSUMPTION OF HIGH-CALORIE ANIMAL PROTEIN.

The honest reason for this dietary change is that the predominant portion of animal protein fed to children is much too calorically dense for their body weight. The typical protein sources given to children are derived from hamburgers, hot dogs, fried chicken, pork chops, and luncheon meats. One of the goals of successful weight loss is to reduce your child's calories without subtracting volume from their daily food intake. This can be easily accomplished by making a couple of protein substitutions. Once you take the time to write down your child's typical food intake for a week, it will be obvious where the excess calories are coming from. The reason I ask you to write down what your child is eating when they are not on a diet is to recognize the foods that are contributing the most calories toward their daily caloric total. If, for instance, your child eats 4,000 calories in a day, and 2,000 of them are from animal protein, you need to reduce the source of these calories.

It's time to play diet detective and determine the actual calories your child derives from animal protein. Let's look at an actual example from a diet client.

food giants decided to add artificial flavors to food so that your body would yearn for more, which in turn increases their sales!

The reason it's essential to give your child a natural multivitamin is to keep them fulfilled and content while dieting. When you look at their diet journal, it becomes obvious that your child doesn't receive enough nutrients, and the simple solution is to give them their vitamins on a daily basis.

11. TEACH YOUR CHILD TO SLOW DOWN WHEN THEY EAT. THEY'RE NOT IN A RACE.

In America, the term "fast" was inserted into a whole category of food. Fast food has earned the title in a justifiable manner. It seems like people in this country are in such a hurry to finish their meal that they aren't taking the time to enjoy their food, and it becomes a way of eating that lends itself to weight gain. The perfect example is the typical family that stops at a fast-food restaurant on their way to do some shopping at the mall. It's rather chilly outdoors, so Mom decides to use the drive-thru window and keep the family cozy and warm inside the vehicle. The children shout their orders out to Mom, who has to make some quick decisions because the order person is asking her to please make her selections, and there are five other vehicles behind them with more hungry children waiting to order. In a matter of minutes, the family car is filled with white bags and cardboard containers with piping hot steam escaping from them, as they are torn open. The drinks are being distributed to their appropriate recipients, and there are condiment packages being passed around the vehicle. The parking lot is practically full, and Mom doesn't feel like waiting for the suitable space, so she decides to drive to the mall and eat on the way there, which saves the family time. In an effort to conserve our nation's most endangered resource: *time*, we have sacrificed our enjoyment of food and the family bonding that occurs when we share our meals together. The results of eating on the run have taken their toll on our society in the form of weight gain.

It's actually an American custom to eat so fast that you don't even recall the actual pleasure that can be derived from eating in a relaxed way. In other parts of the world, dining is a serious matter. In France, the local shops close down for two hours so that the workers can enjoy a peaceful and leisurely lunch. It's a European custom to have several courses at their evening meal, which lasts up to three hours. In other cultures mealtime is a social event in which families come together to share the events of the day and articulate their views and feelings regarding the rest of the world. It's a fact that civilizations that take the time to assemble the family and eat in a relaxed, social manner tend to weigh less. They are not so focused on the race to clean their plate or finish the food in the bag; instead they use food as a context for socialization. They appreciate the meal because it provides them with quality time that they can share with relatives and friends. If all you think about when you eat is how quickly you should devour your food, then you need to look at mealtime in a whole new light.

It's obvious that there are numerous benefits to dining together as a family unit, but if your schedules don't lend themselves to this happening on a nightly basis in your household, then at least try to gather the family together once a week for a true dining experience.

The speed at which your children eat is determined by their parents' influence. If you gobble down your food in a matter of minutes, then your child will tend to mimic your behavior, because that's the only way they've been shown to eat their food. The predominant reason that you need to teach your child to eat slowly is that it takes 10–20 minutes for your brain to know you have food in your stomach. This means that when your child eats a bag of potato chips in 10 minutes, they've consumed 1,500 calories, and their brain doesn't even know they've eaten yet. Therefore, the sensation of fullness hasn't occurred, and their brain doesn't tell their body that they should stop eating.

It's crucial to dieting success that your child feel full both mentally and physically. The first key to this endeavor is to serve food in lesser portions by utilizing the *small plate theory*, as explained earlier. The whole concept of the idea is to reduce the amount of your serving by using a plate that is smaller in size than your usual serving dish. This not only establishes a new reference for portion size; it also slows down the process of eating. It's mentally appealing to look at that full plate because now you can consume all the food on your dish without pangs of guilt. If the serving size of your plate is reduced by half, then the calories are also decreased as a result. The small plate theory saves enough calories that your dieting child can have second portions, which are normally forbidden on most weight loss programs.

The second method of slowing down your child's eating rate is to serve food that takes time to eat. The chewing sensation is an important part of dietary satisfaction. The foods that best fit this category are raw fruits and vegetables. I understand that this type of cuisine does not rank high on most adolescents' favorite food list, but this is generally due to poor presentation and bad eating habits, which are a result of consuming high-calorie junk food. The first step toward convincing your child to eat fruits and vegetables is to have them readily available. If you just throw a bag of carrots and a bunch of grapes in your refrigerator, it's not very appetizing and requires preparation prior to consumption, which puts a damper on the option right from the start. The best way to encourage your child to eat fruits and vegetables is to prepare them in advance and provide delicious condiments to enhance their flavor. Cut up carrots, broccoli, green peppers, and cucumbers and put them in an appetizer tray with a low-calorie ranch dip, which transforms vegetables into a party platter. Then your child can reach into the refrigerator and eat them for a healthy snack. The same trick applies to sprucing up your fruit. The favorable method of serving fruit is to wash and slice such items as grapes, apples, cherries, blueberries, strawberries, and watermelon and to put them on a platter with a low-calorie vanilla yogurt, diet chocolate syrup, or light whipped cream.

There are numerous low-calorie condiments that are suitable to accompany fruits and vegetables, and you should incorporate them into your child's diet according to their individual tastes and preferences. The objective here is to feed your child food that takes time to chew and eat, instead of products that are smooth or mushy, which are swallowed and consumed in a hurried manner. There are plenty of foods that fit these criteria, and the longer it takes to actually eat them, the higher the levels of satisfaction and fullness that result. Do remember to set a good example for your children by eating in a relaxed and slow manner yourself. This way your family can enjoy their food together and share a pleasant conversation at the same time.

12. DETER YOUR DIETING CHILD FROM EATING 500 CALORIES OR MORE IN ONE SITTING.

By decreasing the calories of your child's meals and snacks, you reduce the total daily caloric intake. You also prevent eating episodes that involve a rapid consumption of high-calorie food, which leads to habits that result in obesity. If your child becomes accustomed to consuming too many calories at once, they tend to eat far too many calories by the end of the day. If for instance they're up to their caloric limit for the day by noon, you can't really expect your child to just fast for the rest of the day. It's similar to the old adage of putting all your eggs in one basket. You don't want your child to consume their entire calories for the day in one meal, because you know they will still want to continue eating the rest of their meals. This in turn raises their caloric intake above what's required for weight loss.

Downsizing the per-meal calories also dissuades the consumption of food that's high in caloric density. These foods are usually high in fat and contain artificial flavors, which gets your child's taste buds into the mode of overeating. These types of products are usually referred to as junk food because they are essentially devoid of nutrients, which also leaves your child wanting more! I've always told my clients, "You crave what you eat." Therefore, the sooner you feed your child lower calorie cuisine, the quicker their preferences for these types of food will occur.

If you simply remove 100 calories from breakfast, 200 from lunch, 300 from dinner, and 200 from snacks, you will have saved them 800 calories per day. Don't let your children get themselves into the habit of eating a tremendous amount of calories in one sitting. If they eat a pint of high-calorie ice cream, it will add up to 1,200 calories, all of which can be consumed in a matter of minutes. Then what will they eat the rest of the day? If you discover that your child eats an average of three snacks per day, and each one of them has about 1,500 calories, then they're wasting 4,500 calories per day. If you reduce their snack calories to 500, they'll be saving 3,000 calories per day, which will negate 21,000 calories per week.

TAKING CHARGE

It's the small changes over time that determines the rate of your child's weight loss. It's paramount to your child's diet program that you take the time to write down what they eat on a daily basis, adding up their total caloric intake each day in order to guarantee that they receive the results they deserve. If your child is mature enough to write down what they eat, then by all means *have them do it themselves.* This will teach them a lifelong dietary lesson and provide them with the necessary knowledge to stay a normal weight for their entire life. Once your adolescent is aware that excess calories lead to weight gain, they can make the proper substitutions in order to lose weight without starving, resorting to fad diets, or trying foolish weight loss schemes.

The whole issue of childhood obesity has the country in an uproar, but there seems to be more talking than acting upon the problem at the present time. It's easy to write an article recommending that you increase your child's consumption of fruits and vegetables and raise their level of exercise in order to help your child to lose weight. Then again, the author of these commentaries probably doesn't have a clue about how difficult it can be to drastically change your child's eating habits. It's amazing to find out that the majority of these so-called weight loss experts have never successfully counseled a child and taught them how to lose weight on a one-to-one basis in a real-life situation. You can write volumes about the benefits of a perfectly balanced nutrition program, but it's pointless unless a child can actually live on it.

As a parent, you know your child's likes and dislikes, which means you're the best candidate to be their diet coach. *It's your responsibility to teach your child* how to count their net calories, because this is the only proven scientific method of weight loss in the world! It's not fair to lead your child down a diet path that results in frustration or starvation. That is what happens when you stray from the truth and try to put your child on the latest fad diet. The road to thinness is paved with gold when you follow the laws of science and teach your child to become accountable for the calories they consume each day.

The same principles of dieting apply to both children and adults. The same methods you learn in this book for your own weight loss should be utilized for your child. The main goal is to calculate how many calories they can consume in order to lose weight and adjust their caloric intake accordingly.

If your child is at a point where they're gaining weight on a regular basis, then just maintaining their current weight is equivalent to weight loss and should be considered an accomplishment. This sometimes sounds like an oxymoron to the rookie dieter, so here's an example: if your child gained 8 pounds last month, and this month they didn't gain any weight, then they're 8 pounds ahead of their current pace of weight gain. In other words, your child weighs 8 pounds less than if they didn't diet. This is construed as weight loss and a step in the right direction, which means they are no longer on their way up.

The most pressing issue surrounding childhood obesity is that it results in health problems and life-threatening diseases. *This leads to a sense of urgency about teaching your child how to lose weight.* The sooner you instill lower calorie eating habits, the quicker they become a way of life for your children and the entire family.

In closing, the main priority is to teach your child how to lose weight now! It's a serious matter, and it isn't something you can put off until later or hope they will grow out of. The longer you wait, the more your child will weigh, and this will only extend the amount of time they'll need to diet in order to achieve a healthy body weight. When you instill good dieting habits in your child, you can put your mind at ease this evening, knowing that what you're doing for them will help enrich their lives forever!

15. CHEERS

The most ignored 70 percent of the human body is the percentage of your actual cellular structure that's comprised of water. We've all been told to drink 6 to 8 eight-ounce glasses of it daily to keep healthy, but few of us ever achieve the required allotment. Water is one of the six nutrients necessary to sustain life, yet it's often the most neglected aspect of our daily intake. So let's take a look at the myths that have been perpetuated in regards to this elixir of life.

The most common of these dietary myths is that all fluids are created equal. Every diet book instructs you to drink plenty of water in order to stimulate weight loss, yet many dieters ignore the rules and substitute other liquids for water. It's a scientific fact that in a laboratory you never use anything but distilled water for a chemical experiment. You can't use tap water because it can contain up to 700 chemicals, which will react with the other substances that the scientist is using in their chemical equations. The point I'm making is simple. There is no known liquid on earth that will substitute for distilled water in the human body. You're only cheating yourself when you count the coffee, tea, and soda you drink as part of your water requirement.

The second myth is that it's better to drink spring water than distilled water. This rumor started when the lay public thought that somehow the human body could utilize the inorganic minerals in spring water, which is scientifically and biologically impossible! The inorganic minerals in spring water can collect on the lining of your arteries and lead to arteriosclerosis. The human body can only utilize organic minerals like those contained in fruits and vegetables, so do your health a favor and switch from spring water to distilled water, which is the superior choice.

If distilled water is unavailable and you must choose between spring water and tap water, the logical choice is spring water. The mere fact that tap water could cause thousands of illnesses a year is reason enough to keep it where it belongs: in the toilet, not in your glass. That leads me to the third misunderstanding regarding water:

Most Americans think that tap water is safe and healthy for daily consumption. They assume that their local water processing facility has redeemed the water by adding chlorine, which is harmful to your health. Let's take a look at some of the most common harmful substances found in tap water:

Radon	Lead	Fertilizers	Chlorine
Fluoride	Copper	Asbestos	Carbon
Arsenic	Chloroform	Cyanides	Lime
Iron	Heavy Metals	Herbicides	Soda Ash
Pesticides	Parasites	Industrial Chemicals	Aluminum Sulfate
Bacteria	Viruses		

In a study conducted by the Natural Resources Defense Council, they found that 18,500 of our nation's water systems violated the safe drinking water laws. These water systems provide 45 million Americans with unsafe tap water! The high levels of chlorine and fluoride are two prominent reasons not to gulp down tap water. It is a well-known fact that the chlorine byproducts in tap water are toxic to the human body and accumulate in fatty tissue, body fat, and mother's milk. The addition of chlorine to water increases the risk of several forms of cancer and can contribute to the onset of heart disease.

One of the most controversial events ever to happen on a national scale was the decision to add fluoride to drinking water. In 1961, the Congressional Record exposed fluoride as a lethal poison! The original scheme was to proclaim to the public that adding fluoride to their water would reduce the incidence of tooth decay and cavities. Yet there has never been any scientific proof that fluoride helps to prevent tooth decay. In fact, numerous reputable studies have proven the opposite. In 1955, the original promoter of water fluoridation even admitted under oath that it doesn't work as a remedy for tooth decay. It's a well-known fact that fluoride damages the teeth and weakens the bones. There is a multitude of evidence that proves fluoride is unsafe for human consumption. The main reason it was put into water in the first place was to dispose of fluoride wastes. In 1939, there were 45 industries that were trying to lower the cost of disposing their fluoride waste products, and they decided to come up with a brilliant plan. The idea was to dissolve the fluoride into the drinking water and be paid by the government to do so, instead of chemical companies having to pay to get rid of their toxic wastes. They led the public to believe that they were doing them a favor by tainting their water supply with poison! The results were devastating, but the power of corporate America kept the truth from the public. Listed below are some of the various health problems caused by consuming fluoride.

Osteoporosis	Genetic damage
Learning disabilities	Osteofluorosis
Neurological impairment	Hip fractures
Lower IQ in children	Nausea
Deformities	Vomiting
Acceleration of tumor growth	Diarrhea
Irreparable harm to the immune system	Fertility problems
Reduced resistance to infection	
Damages teeth and tooth enamel	

For dieting the best possible choice for water consumption is distilled water for several reasons. It's important to re-hydrate your body with pure water in order to detoxify your system and expedite weight loss. The best-known way to clean and purify every cell and organ in the human body is by drinking distilled water. This is turn will stimulate your body to process the food you eat more efficiently and boost your metabolism because the body is able to absorb and transport vital nutrients on a cellular level. It's a fact that drinking distilled water stimulates weight loss and is referred to as the single most significant factor that determines permanent weight loss. It's interesting to note that Hollywood movie stars have been drinking it in order to retain their youthful looks. The distilled water prevents dehydration and keeps the body's cells healthier. As a result, the face and neck remain free of aging lines and wrinkles, because the distilled water helps stop the skin from wrinkling and leaves it clear and healthy.

There are so many health benefits from drinking distilled water that several books have been published on the topic. If you care to expand your water horizons, I suggest you read Paul Bragg's book, simply titled *Water*. The next time you fill your glass, do your diet and health a favor, and make your next toast with distilled water. *Salud!*

TOP TEN REASONS WHY WATER ENCOURAGES WEIGHT LOSS

1. Water transports nutrients to various locations in the body. Therefore, the increased absorption of your vitamins and minerals decreases your appetite.

2. Water removes toxins from the body. This enables your liver to work more efficiently at eliminating excess fat from the body.

3.   Water is essential to proper digestion. When digestion is more efficient, you absorb fewer calories, which in turn results in quicker weight loss.

4.   Water provides a feeling of fullness, which in turn reduces hunger.

5.   Water hydrates the cells of the body, which prevents fluid retention, bloating, and weight gain.

6.   Water increases your metabolism by removing excess waste and toxins from your body.

7.   Water helps to maintain your muscle tone. Therefore, you're able to maintain a sleek, trim body.

8.   Water cleanses the palate and quenches thirst better than any other beverage.

9.   Water contains zero calories, which is perfect for a dieter. There are numerous varieties of water on the market today such as seltzers and flavored types that are calorie free and taste great.

10. Water is an important catalyst in losing weight and keeping it off.

16. SALT CITY

This is not a mythological town in some fantasy movie. It's actually the nick-name of my hometown, Syracuse, New York. It's a city well versed in the attributes of salt. In fact, our school took each class on a fieldtrip to explore the salt museum. The art of deriving salt from the earth was described in detail, as we peered at what looked like the world's largest salt wheel.

There are plenty of rumors that swirl around the diet industry, and perhaps one of the most common myths about dieting concerns the consumption of salt. It's a typical scene in the diet food aisle of the grocery store when you overhear the conversation of a rookie dieter trying to select the proper diet cuisine. "I like soy sauce on my rice, but it's got too much sodium for me. So perhaps I'll just use butter instead, or have it plain." Let's examine the mistakes made by this dieter:

Mistake #1:   Omit salt to lose weight.

Mistake #2:   Replace salt with butter to lose weight

Mistake #3:   Replace salt with butter to reduce your sodium intake.

Mistake #4:   Eat your food plain, which makes it bland and boring, just because you're trying to avoid salt-laden condiments.

The primary reason diets discourage the use of salt is because of water retention. If you drastically reduce your consumption of salt your first week of dieting, it appears as though your weight drops rapidly. This in turn gives you a false sense of diet security, because you start to think that you can keep up this pace of weight loss on a weekly basis. Then all of a sudden you consume foods that are higher in sodium than the items on their specific menu program, and you gain weight. You then become discouraged and wonder what has happened to your successful weight loss. You start to blame other factors such as yourself, when in fact it was just a fluid fluctuation caused by an increase of sodium in your diet. The scale doesn't differentiate between fluid, bone, and muscle; it just registers your total body mass.

There are several reasons salt has been given a bum rap in the Unites States. The foremost of these is that when scientists process and refine salt, it becomes sodium chloride, not real salt from the earth. The product is raised to high temperatures, and chemical anti-caking agents are added for the consumer's convenience. It's one of those cases where science intervenes and decides to produce a purely chemical replacement in order to increase their profit margin.

There is plenty of confusion over the salt issue because most consumers are told it causes hypertension (high blood pressure). There are several risk factors that contribute to high blood pressure, and obesity is the primary reason for the disease. Therefore, weight loss is the most logical way to lower your blood pressure. I have had numerous clients say that after losing weight, they no longer have hypertension. Let me give you a perfect example of such a dieter. His name is Ralph. When he started dieting, Ralph's weight was 204 pounds, and his blood pressure was 130/95. When he reached his weight loss goal, he weighed 164 pounds, and his blood pressure dropped to 110/68. The only dietary change he made pertaining to sodium was to eat sea salt instead of conventional table salt. Ralph's blood pressure was reduced by 47 points because of his lower body weight. He has maintained his weight loss and continues to use sea salt to this day.

The issue that concerns me about drastically decreasing your sodium intake is the fact that it's not a livable concept. If this method of dieting were successful, then why is hypertension on the rise? It's increasing because obesity rates are higher. The average person will not stay on a sodium-free diet for the rest of their life, and therefore they need other options that they can actually commit to and achieve noticeable results. Ask yourself how long you could live on a bland diet.

The first problem with negating salt from your diet is that food becomes boring and tasteless unless you take the time to spice up your recipes with herbs and spices. If you become disgruntled with the flavor of your food, it's difficult to adhere to your dietary program. The best diet program is the one you can live with and benefit from on a daily basis.

The second obstacle that occurs when dieters try to eliminate salt is what they choose to replace the sodium. It's a common fallacy that it's acceptable to add condiments like butter or oil instead of salt. This is a dietary disaster when you take a look at the consequences of such a decision. It's never logical to replace salt with fat, because salt has no calories, and fat has 240 calories per ounce. This mistake could cause a weight gain of 25 pounds each year if you used only one ounce of fat per day instead of salt.

The reality of the situation is that most dieters will not give up salt, and you shouldn't have to in order to lose weight. The real issue is how to make the best salt selection.

The most logical way to make a choice is to be armed with the appropriate knowledge. The two main options for salt are what our culture calls table salt (refined salt) or sea salt (unrefined salt). Let's first look at the structural and chemical differences between the two.

Sea Salt	Table Salt
1. Sea salt contains 98% NaCl (Sodium Chloride) and 2% other minerals.	1. Sodium Chloride in its chemical form NaCl is 60.663% Chlorine and 39.337% sodium (Na)
2. Sea salt has over 92 essential minerals, which are comprised of 80 elements.	2. Table salt has been stripped of its additional minerals and elements.
3. Sea salt doesn't have any additives whatsoever.	3. Table salt consists of several additives such as sugar, aluminum, silicate, yellow prussiate of soda, and various bleaches.
4. Sea salt neutralizes toxins and detrimental bacteria in the human body.	4. Refined salt adds toxins to the body, which contribute to various diseases. Aluminum silicate is added to refined salt, which is used to keep it powdery. The aluminum used is a highly toxic chemical that is one of the primary causes of Alzheimer's disease.
5. Sea salt is required for the proper digestion of plant carbohydrates. When sea salt is added to fruits and vegetables, the body secretes saliva and gastric juices, which in turn break down the fibrous portion of carbohydrates.	5. Refined salt does not have the ability to perpetuate the digestion of plant carbohydrates and causes thirst upon indigestion. The desire for fluids is a sign of being poisoned. Therefore, fibrous foods such as fruits, vegetables, and grains are not being assimilated fully. This in turn depletes the body of essential nutrients.
6. Because sea salt provides the body with essential minerals, it's satisfying both mentally and physically.	6. The consumption of refined salt causes a craving for more salt because it depletes the body of vital minerals.
7. Sea salt is dried naturally by the sun.	7. Refined salt is raised to extremely high temperatures, which destroys its molecular structure, thereby nullifying its nutritional content.
8. Sea salt balances the amount of water that stays outside the body's cells.	8. Refined salt causes water imbalances, which in turn results in chronic kidney problems.
9. Sea salt enhances calcium absorption and helps the body to absorb the nutrients.	9. Refined salt interferes with the absorption of nutrients and depletes the body of calcium.

After reviewing the above chart, it's obvious that sea salt is the optimum choice when purchasing salt. However, many consumers are confused by the vast array of selections available to them. It's important not to be led astray by ingenious marketing schemes, so let the buyer beware. The one simple rule of thumb when purchasing food products that contain salt is to buy organic food. If an item is organic, FDA law requires any salt in that item to be sea salt. This takes the guesswork out of shopping and saves a lot of label-reading time.

When you purchase salt as a single item, make sure that the label says it is pure sea salt and doesn't contain any other ingredients. It's a common misunderstanding that kosher salt is natural, but it's refined just like the other table salts on the market. If regular salt is put in a fancy package at a gourmet shop, it's still refined and thus unhealthy.

Remember, you can have your sea salt and eat it too, without guilt or weight gain!

17. BACK IN THE SADDLE AGAIN

(For those thinking about quitting)

TOP TEN REASONS WHY I CAN'T STAY ON A DIET

1. "THAT DIET DIDN'T WORK FOR ME!"

I've had to make rebuttals to this statement for two decades. The answer is simple. Was the diet even worth trying in the first place? You must expend more calories than you consume in order to lose weight. So first, you must know how many net calories you eat per day in order to logically answer your question. If you don't know how many calories you eat, and you're not responsible for your food intake, then to put it quite simply: you're not dieting! The math behind weight loss is based on your current weight and the amount of calories it takes to maintain that weight. No one goes against the laws of science, so use them to your advantage. The good news is that if you haven't started a real diet yet, then the best part is learning how to genuinely control your caloric intake and enjoy your life at the same time.

2. "I DON'T HAVE TIME TO WRITE DOWN WHAT I EAT!"

I would normally respond to this by saying, "You certainly found the time to eat." Think of all the things we find time to do when we want to do them. People spend time on their hair and makeup every morning, and others even fit in trips to the hairstylist and squeeze nail tip appointments into their busy schedule. It takes me less than five minutes to write down what I eat every day. That is less than the required time of a break at work. Now even the busiest dieter can use their work break in a productive manner.

3. "I HAVE A SLOW METABOLISM, SO DIETS DON'T WORK FOR ME."

My first replies will always be, "Do you know how many calories you eat each day?" and "Did you keep a food journal?" Then the most common answers I've heard in 20 years are, "No, I don't know how many calories I eat," and "No, I don't keep a diary." Well, you won't know whether you have a fast or slow metabolism until you find out how many calories it takes to maintain your weight. Even if it turns out that you have a snail-like metabolism like I do, this will be the perfect diet for you. I will teach you how to eat more and weigh less while boosting your metabolism permanently!

4. "I DON'T EAT MUCH AT ALL, BUT I STILL CAN'T SEEM TO LOSE WEIGHT."

The problem here is the definition of a small portion of food. Foods with a high caloric density don't take much; they quickly add up and put you over your daily caloric limit. If you eat foods with a low caloric density, then you'll still be safe even if your estimate of portion size is a little off. If I think I ate one cup of green beans but I really had 1½ cups, I'll only be off by 12.5 calories. However, if I thought a restaurant put only one tablespoons of high-calorie olive oil on my salad, when in fact they put on four, then I'm off by 360 calories. If you make an error like this ten times in one week, you'll end up gaining a pound even though you're on a diet.

I tell my clients that you must measure when it comes to fats. If you're willing to give up other food in order to eat fats, then you sacrifice volume. I suggest that you consume food that can be chewed, tasted, and appreciated b so that you feel full and satisfied. Learn to experiment with spices and low-calorie condiments as an alternative to oil, butter, and margarine. Since fats don't contribute any flavor to the recipe, don't waste the calories. If you were eating as little as you thought, then you wouldn't have gained weight in the first place. When it comes to fats, it only takes a little to gain weight.

5. "MY FAMILY DOESN'T LIKE DIET FOODS!"

The answer here lies in the presentation. How we perceive something will determine our reaction. There are plenty of makeover shows hitting the airwaves with great success. Everyone loves to see an ordinary woman transformed into a beautiful model. It's exciting to watch a hut turned into a mansion. This is exactly what you need to do to your diet meals. If your family doesn't like the food, it's because your recipes need a makeover.

You would be surprised how many children will devour a pasta casserole with veggies baked into it because they take on the flavor of the tomato sauce. I tell my clients to incorporate their fruits and vegetables into their recipe. Casseroles and one-pot meals are wonderful dietary cooking options the whole family can enjoy. This is just one simple example of how nutritious food can be used to make any recipe a low-calorie recipe.

I wouldn't expect a family to enjoy lettuce in a bowl with low-calorie dressing, so instead design a taco bar and have the family build their meal together. This way you can have onions, tomatoes, and lettuce with all the flavor and spices, and they will enjoy their vegetables.

You need to call a family meeting and have everyone write down their five favorite fruits and their five favorite vegetables. This gives you a reference point. For instance, if we know that everyone in the family likes corn, you can use it in your diet meals.

You need to instill proper eating habits for the whole family because you don't want your children to end up overweight. If they eat the food that made you overweight, they're bound to gain weight as well. If they're already overweight, then there's no better time than now to start teaching them how to lose weight. The longer you wait, the more they'll weigh!

6. "I FEEL HUNGRY EVERY TIME I DIET!"

Then you're on the wrong diet. There are plenty of obnoxious programs that expect you to consume 800 or fewer calories per day. I've seen menu programs that wouldn't satisfy a hamster let alone a human. I invented recipes that are so large, my dieters have told me it takes them a whole week to eat one diet recipe. I've prepared pasta casseroles that weigh 8 pounds and contain only 1,200 calories. Guests who eat at my social gatherings have told me that they're so full, they don't even want to eat the next day until mid-afternoon. I feel sorry for dieters that adhere to low volume menu programs, because they could be having an all-you-can-eat dinner every night on this program and still wake up thinner the next morning!

7. "I DON'T HAVE THE WILLPOWER TO STAY ON A DIET! I TEND TO CHEAT WHEN I'M DENIED CERTAIN FOODS."

You won't need willpower to stay on this diet because it's designed by you, for you. You can format a menu that's personalized specifically to fulfill your dietary needs. I'm not going to tell you what to eat; instead, I'll teach you how to eat the foods you enjoy and lose weight at the same time. When you're armed with the proper dietary knowledge, you don't need willpower; you need to make the right choices. Simple changes in your diet over a period of time will yield permanent weight loss.

8. "MY PROFESSION INVOLVES A LOT OF TRAVEL, AND I EAT OUT REGULARLY, SO I CAN'T STAY ON A DIET BECAUSE OF MY SCHEDULE."

Even if traveling is required, poor eating is not. You can choose to travel and be overweight or travel and be normal weight. You need to determine that weight loss is your goal and then alter your food intake according to your individual situation. You obviously pass plenty of health food shops and grocery stores on your travels, and you should stop in for a quick and nutritious meal. Plan your schedule ahead of time and map out your trip so you can eat out in restaurants that will accommodate your dietary requests.

9. "I DON'T EAT A BALANCED DIET, AND I SKIP MEALS. IT'S DIFFICULT FOR ME TO STAY ON A SPECIFIC REGIMEN."

That's fine, because neither do I. This diet was invented to break the traditional dietary rules and still help you lose weight. I have counseled clients for two decades, and I've never seen a dieter eat a perfectly balanced diet. You eat when you want to eat. I detest programs that tell me how many meals you have to eat, or diets that tell me I can't eat at night. These types of programs are so strict, they're like having a drill sergeant on your back, compelling you to adhere to the rules and regulations. The one and only simple rule you need to follow is to be responsible for what you consume.

10. "I'VE BEEN OVERWEIGHT SINCE I WAS A CHILD. NO DIET HAS EVER WORKED FOR ME. I GUESS I'M DOOMED TO BE FAT FOR THE REST OF MY LIFE."

The first step you need to take is to change your attitude. Your eating habits are what got you into this situation in the fist place. That's excellent news because habits are a learned behavior. It's now up to you to change these bad habits into good habits. *There is not one person on earth who is doomed to be overweight.* This program will teach you how to make small changes in order to promote permanent weight loss. It's important to get started immediately because once you start losing weight, your frame of mind will change. *I can help anyone in the world lose weight if they just determine that it's something they really want to do!*

THE BINGE

It happens before you even realize it. All of a sudden, you've consumed your daily caloric intake in a single sitting, but it's the aftermath that's the worst part of the whole situation. There's the guilt, and then comes the punishment. We're taught as children that there are consequences to doing something wrong, and our brain goes into the mode of discipline. Most programs make us feel like a failure and thus cause us to quit before we even have a chance to succeed, but there is valuable information to be learned about oneself from this experience: it's not as bad as it seems. The first question you should ask yourself is, "How much would I have consumed if I weren't on a diet?" If you're eating less than you would have, then you're stepping forward in a positive direction.

Why a dieter binges can be broken down into three levels. I call them 1st, 2nd, and 3rd degree binges. A binge is by definition an act of overeating that contributes to weight gain and results in a feeling of remorse and guilt. A third degree binge is the lowest level of an eating frenzy. This occurs when you plan on following your diet and someone brings you bad food or serves you high-calorie food. Even after all your good intentions, you find yourself eating the food you promised yourself you would not. A second-degree binge is when you wake up in the morning and plan on following your diet. You are called into a meeting, and they have donuts. Now you eat the donut because you see the donut. A second-degree binge occurs when you eat food because you see the food. A first-degree binge is the supreme diet crime. It calls for punishment by the diet police. This is the case where you actually planned the binge. It's a case of premeditated eating. You planned it, then you bought the food, and you ate it. This means you were fully aware of the impending doom, yet you did it anyway.

Being responsible for what you eat is one of the key factors to your success. One of my 370-pound clients put it to me candidly. He (Bill) stated that every day was like Thanksgiving to him. I replied, "What if you changed that to every other day, and you could still lose weight. Wouldn't that be better than your current situation?" He agreed and proceeded to change his habits in small increments. What he needed to do was set himself up for success, not failure.

When you first embark on your weight loss program, it's very important to allow yourself leeway to make changes or mistakes. If you set unattainable goals, you don't prosper. If a marathon runner had to do 26 miles the first time he ever ran, I'm sure he wouldn't do it again, so if you start out your first week by trying to lose 10 pounds, and you don't, then naturally you'll be tempted to say, "Forget this diet."

As each action has an equal and opposite reaction in the world of science, so it does in the diet world. The binge is a reaction to something, so you need to identify which action led up to it. Then you'll be forewarned next time.

I'll give you a typical circumstance that could result in an unplanned binge. I'm sure you've heard the phrase "birds of a feather flock together." I quote that because it's what pops into my mind after so many years of hearing "binge" and "pig out" stories. People eat in group situations such as birthday parties or weddings. Now take yourself out of the picture and look upon yourself as a spectator when people are assembled into groups; they do things out of peer pressure. Why do dieters have to go out only to come home with tremendous pangs of guilt and sometimes give up their diet, all because of one setback? Isn't it possible to stand firm against social pressures and eat as you choose? Yes, it is!

I'll give you an example from my own life. As far back as I can remember I knew that birthday cake was unhealthy for me. Both my grandparents were diabetic, and my three aunts were each over 250 pounds. The one thing I was sure of was that I didn't want to look like them. Therefore, I knew I wasn't going to eat what they ate. I don't remember ever eating a piece of my own birthday cake. Actually, I was lucky in a way, because the original reason that I did it was a result of my grandparents' diabetes. I would tell my family that if grandma and grandpa couldn't eat the cake, neither would I. My family said that I was ruining the party, so I obviously understand peer pressure. When you take yourself outside the picture and look upon yourself as a spectator, you'll see these social situations in a new light. Are you really going there to celebrate a birthday or to eat cake and ice cream?

I was discussing the peer pressure of eating with my husband, and he said there was one statement he remembered since he met me (23 years ago) that he would never forget. He still vividly recalls what I said at the party. When I was told to go ahead, live it up, enjoy myself, eat what everyone else was eating because they didn't want me to be left out, I told him, *"No one can make me eat what I don't want to!"* That would just make me feel guilty.

Now, I'm a bit confused, I said to myself. *I'm not supposed to feel guilty when I binge with a group of people while I'm doing it, and then when it's over I'm supposed to feel guilty?* It's that guilty after-thought that gets us on the path to dieting disasters. I should have said setbacks here, but I've seen it lead to worse. An example of an actual diet client will explain it all. This person came home from a party and started thinking, *oh well, I've really blown that diet today, so why not continue eating and start again tomorrow?* The thing to remember is that a diet is about the total calories eaten over the long run, not just one day. Everyone makes mistakes, so why continue to punish yourself? It's time to remind yourself that the goal here is to lose weight, not gain it. It's important to think of how it will make you feel if you gain weight.

Will you then quit the diet completely and go right back to your old eating habits? What will that accomplish but more guilt? In psychiatric terms, this behavior would be called circular reasoning. Just remember it takes one line to make a circle, and it doesn't end, does it? Here's a diagram of a dieter using circular reasoning to justify their actions:

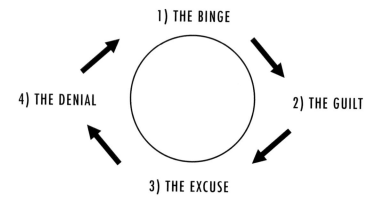

1) THE BINGE

4) THE DENIAL

2) THE GUILT

3) THE EXCUSE

1. I went to a social event and binged.

2. I felt guilty and developed a self-defeating impulse to give up, so I continued the binge.

3. Now I think I've gained weight, so why not just give that diet a rest for a while? After all, I didn't follow it anyway.

4. I just can't seem to lose weight, so why not just eat and enjoy myself?

It's simple to turn all this into positive behavior. Following a binge, just recognize that you did it; it's done; now forget about it and go on. Don't let it stand in your way of getting thin. The sooner you forgive yourself, the quicker you'll achieve your weight loss goal. Concentration on a goal always takes a step forward, not backward. This is much easier than you think, and it helps us prepare ourselves mentally for the next temptation that might arise!

WHAT'S MY BONUS?

Each person has a specific motivation to stay on a diet program, and I always tell my clients that it should be a motivation that speaks to you personally. Well, here's the best incentive known to mankind: *The latest scientific research on caloric restriction indicates that reducing your calories is the best way to increase your life span!* An article published in the *Scientific American* stated that the best longevity strategy is to decrease your caloric intake. The scientists agreed that a reduced calorie diet was absolutely proven to work for prolonging healthy longevity. It's comforting to know that such a simple thing as reducing your caloric intake will add years onto your life. That's what I call a bonus, because if you really think about it, the payoff far exceeds the effort.

The scientists also found several health bonuses from the reduction of calories. These benefits will provide a multitude of motivations to stay on your diet:

1. Heart health is significantly improved.

    *   It prevents aging of the heart.

    *   There's a reduction in the total cholesterol and LDL levels.

    *   There's a rise in the artery-protective lipoprotein HDL.

    *   Your heart has a "powerful protective effect against atherosclerosis."

    *   A rejuvenating effect occurs on the heart and overall health.

2. The brain is healthier. Scientists were amazed at the results. They concluded that cutting back on calories not only enables our brains to remain healthy, it improves our memory.

3. Caloric restriction helps prevent common diseases. After only five weeks of lowering their caloric intake, the participants' blood pressure readings were substantially lowered, and so were their cholesterol levels. The significance of reducing blood pressure and cholesterol is primarily related to decreasing your risk of developing cardiovascular diseases. The mere act of eating fewer calories can help prevent you from getting a stroke or heart attack.

4. Insulin levels are lowered. In a recent study of subjects that reduced their calories for six months, they determined that this type of dieting significantly decreased insulin levels. This is of major importance because high insulin levels are dangerous to the human body, since they result in high blood pressure. Another problem regarding increased insulin is that it can encourage the progression of cancer, and the most obvious outcome of high insulin levels is diabetes. Therefore reducing your calories is the best way to help prevent the disease.

5. The immune system is stimulated. This is advantageous to good health and longevity because disease and illness all stem from a compromised immune system, and when you feel good, it's much easier to exercise and continue with your diet program.

6. Reducing your calories slows down the human aging process. Now that's a bonus that far exceeds the effort.

7. Here's one more bonus: you'll look better. The best way to lower your body fat is by reducing your calories. When the fat is reduced, your muscles appear more clearly defined, so your body looks more toned.

It's also paramount to longevity that you reduce your body fat. The main reason is that toxins house themselves in fat cells. Therefore, the higher your body fat, the more space your toxins have to live in. Fat cells also produce chemicals called cytokines that in turn cause inflammation. This condition eventually leads to cardiovascular disease, heart attacks, and strokes. The motive to reduce your body fat is that it's imperative to good health.

Any time you consider backsliding or quitting your diet program, get yourself back on track by contemplating all the bonuses that a healthy diet gives you each and every day!

FOR THE LADIES

If you're still debating whether to continue your weight loss program, there's another advantage, which concerns the ladies. It's regarding the journey in a woman's life from menses to menopause. I've owned a natural food store for over ten years. This has given me ample time to hear the horror stories regarding menopause symptoms. I would listen intently, wondering if this was my impending fate. Before I opened the store, I looked forward to the time when my menses would cease. Prior to menopause, a reduced-calorie diet affects your menses. When you lower your body fat, the body produces less estrogen, which in turn allows your body to function more efficiently. In turn, the words premenstrual syndrome (PMS) will soon be eliminated from your vocabulary. I used to joke about my menses to my clients, saying that if I didn't write down the date of my monthly period, I wouldn't even know when it was coming. The symptoms that plague menstruating women are a direct result of hormonal imbalance, which is a backlash of having high body fat. As soon as you lower your level of accumulated fat, your body will respond immediately and your premenstrual symptoms will diminish and eventually vanish. It's not normal to have a painfully difficult menses, and you owe it to yourself to experience a pain-free life.

The whole issue of menopause has been blown out of proportion in America. The medical industry actually had the nerve to try to coerce the Food and Drug Administration (FDA) into calling it a disease! The ulterior motive behind this demeaning classification was to increase the sales of hormone replacement drugs and eliminate the natural menopause supplements altogether. The pharmaceutical companies wanted to obliterate their competition in order to increase their profits. The nerve of trying to call menopause a disease is alarming in itself. How can the natural course of a women's life be construed as a disease? In the future, will the medical establishment have the audacity to call aging a disease?

In an overweight person, however, menopause is often accompanied by undesirable symptoms, and their underlying cause is a disease. The United States currently classifies obesity as a disease. According to Webster, the definition of disease is: an alteration of the normal state of the living body that impairs the performance of the vital functions.

The main problem with the American medical system is that it masks symptoms. If you go to a doctor and you're given a prescription drug to suppress your menopause problems, you still haven't addressed the cause of the situation. The underlying reason for your undesirable symptoms is a direct result of being overweight. The excess weight that you carry around incites a hormonal imbalance. The fact that your body is out of equilibrium triggers chemical reactions that eventually show up in the form of hot flashes, night sweats, and mood changes.

The simple and healthy way to transition from menses to menopause is to lose weight. This allows the body to perform at peak condition. You can't appreciate the bonuses of being normal weight until you start losing weight. Other cultures with low rates of obesity don't have the menopause complaints that Americans do.

In my own experience, it's a pleasure to report that the only change in my life was that my menses ceased. After a year without a period, I mentally accepted the fact that I'm menopausal. There wasn't one clue or undesirable symptom during the transition.

This diet program offers better perks than you can fathom. It's your God-given right to be healthy and disease free, but it's up to you to achieve this lifestyle because you have also been granted free will. Your primary goal is to eliminate the first disease, obesity, because good things come to those who are normal weight.

OVER 40, OVERWEIGHT

If this topic describes your current weight status, then don't wait any longer to diet. It's a time in your life when eating additional calories can cause weight gain rather quickly. It's a juncture in your life where the decisions you make will determine your longevity. If you lose weight, your whole quality of life changes, and you won't reap these benefits until you start to diet and experience all the bonuses that go hand in hand with weight loss.

This is the age where excuses often accompany weight gain. It's a time when the body goes through several biochemical changes that lead to a change in bodily functions. It's common knowledge that your metabolism decreases as you age. Yet, most dieters act as if it's only happening to them, like they're being punished by some outside force that only picks on them. It's comforting to know that we're all going through the same mechanisms of aging together. It's more important to adjust your diet according to your body's metabolic requirements than it is to sit around and make excuses why you can't lose weight because you're getting older.

If you think of it logically, excuses are a way to justify our actions. They provide us with an alternative to facing the facts. It's all too common to vindicate our actions in order to continue the behavior. There is another option that you can choose in order to take positive steps toward weight loss. How about taking out a piece of paper and pen and writing down all the reasons why you need to lose weight. What I'm asking you to do is turn a negative into a positive, which is always beneficial toward achieving any goal.

The best way to begin any activity is to establish motives. In this case the activity is dieting, and the motives are based upon your own individual situations and inspirations. If the motivation is strong enough, the goal becomes attainable. One of my lifelong goals was to develop a diet that is perceivable, believable, livable, and achievable. The key here is *able*. You must determine in your mind that you are able to complete the task at hand, which in this case is to lose weight. The difference between a winner and a loser is simply the manner in which they attempt to accomplish their goal.

It's often comforting to justify your actions by saying that everyone else has the problem, so "How can I be any different?" If you use mere numbers as an excuse, then your defense is weak. If you're looking for reasons to be overweight, then you're not in the mode of dieting. It's time to personalize your motive to diet. The purpose of this exercise is to establish the particular reasons why you want to lose weight. It's time to *spark your burning desire* to lose weight. It's the personal motives that will provide the fuel in order to keep the diet fire glowing. Listed below are the top ten reasons why most people start diets. The next section after it illustrates examples of an actual diet client's personalized reasons to start a weight loss program. Next, write down your own personal reasons to diet.

TOP TEN REASONS TO LOSE WEIGHT

1. To live a longer, healthier life.

2. To cure and prevent obesity related diseases (such as high blood pressure, high cholesterol, diabetes, heart disease, etc.).

3. You want to look better and feel good about your appearance.

4. You desire a date and eventually a mate.

5. To alleviate joint, back, and arthritic problems.

6. To fit into your favorite clothes.

7. To attend a particular social event.

8. You want to spice up your marriage.

9. To improve your attitude and mood.

10. You want to be a good example for your children and family to follow.

It's important to rationalize each item in the context of your own life. The initial step toward weight loss must be taken by you, for you. When you're armed with the right ammunition, it's much easier to fight the battle of the bulge. After each reason, take the time to jot down what it personally means to you. It's much easier to diet when you've established the foundation for your plan of action. It's important to remind yourself of the rationale for your weight loss.

Listed below is an example of a completed list of the top ten reasons to diet, written by an actual client.

1. If I don't lose that extra 50 pounds, chances are I won't live to see or enjoy my retirement.

2. I already have high blood pressure and high cholesterol, which is brought on by the extra weight I carry around. When I get back to normal weight, I'll be free of disease and worry.

3. I've been avoiding myself every time I pass a full-length mirror. It's about time I face the facts that I don't even like the way I look anymore.

4. I put on a lot of weight prior to my divorce. It's about time I paid attention to the way I look so that I can get a date.

5. I've gone to physical therapy, chiropractors, and been on drugs for my aches and pains, and I'm still suffering. If I get the extra 50 pounds off my back that I carry around, I'll feel like a new person.

6. I've had that dress in my closet for years because I've always hoped that someday I'll fit back into it. I'm not throwing it away because this time I'm going to wear it to my own birthday party!

7. I'm attending my high school reunion, and I'm not going to be the person they talk about and say, "My, she sure has gained a lot of weight since school. Wasn't she into sports back then?"

8. I sure could use a boost to my romantic relationship with my husband. I can't remember the last time we spent an evening alone together. I'm going to lose weight, buy some new sexy evening attire, and rent the honeymoon suite for the weekend!

9. I can't fit into my clothes anymore, and I refuse to buy larger sizes. I've been snapping at my children lately, and my husband noticed that I'm not the cheerful woman he married. I shouldn't take my weight gain out on my loved ones, but I still do. I'm losing weight so that I'm happy with myself. Then I'll treat the rest of the world a lot nicer when I'm content and satisfied with my own body.

10. It seems as if the whole family has gained weight. We really should stop eating out. I need to stop making excuses for consuming sweets and snacks. If I let the children eat whatever they want, they will just end up as overweight as their parents. I'm going to introduce lower-calorie foods into our family's diet so we can lose weight. I'll start making some gourmet diet recipes and show the family how delicious real food tastes! I need to do something right now before my children develop permanent health problems from their unhealthy eating habits and gain weight.

It's a fact that obesity affects every aspect of your life daily. The good news is that you can make small changes on a daily basis that will alter the current situation. It's important to develop a dieting frame of mind. The beauty of this diet is that you reap the rewards immediately. It's an endeavor that pays off within a day or two. There aren't many things in life that offer instant compensation. When you look at weight loss in the proper perspective, it offers a golden opportunity that can last an entire lifetime! It's time to put aside the excuses and proceed to reap the benefits of this diet. It's important to remember that all the excuses in the world didn't make you thin. The sooner you take responsibility for your food intake, the quicker you will achieve your weight loss goal.

18. STOKE THE FIRE

The most important thing about exercise is to get in the habit. I have told my clients countless times to just walk 10 minutes per day. They tend to reply by saying, "That isn't enough," and I reply, "Well, it's certainly better than not walking at all." The main reason people don't adhere to exercise programs is because they set goals that aren't attainable in their present condition. You don't have to be an Olympian. Just get moving. You basically want to burn calories, which translates to weight loss, but there are more reasons to exercise.

Exercise boosts the metabolism throughout the day. Scientific studies prove that you burn additional calories for up to 8 hours after exercise. So basically, you're adding fuel to the metabolic fire.

It sets up a whole new attitude about yourself. I have heard countless stories of boasting and bragging about the first good workout. No one I know wants to run up a hill huffing, puffing, sweating, and then come home and squander it all by eating a piece of cake. It's just not worth it anymore. After all, you're now part of an elite group. You're among the athletes; you're no longer a couch potato. Perhaps you even find yourself at a sporting goods store, actually shopping for designer sportswear, and all of a sudden you find yourself waving at a fellow walker. The beginning is such a happy time; now stick with it.

Make the program livable. How many of you right now would need to dust off their exercise equipment before they could use it? Like I told my clients, I don't really use my treadmill much because I feel like a hamster in a wheel. You need a kind of exercise you can look forward to. If the exercise equipment was so much fun and so successful, then why don't you look like the person in the commercial yet? Why are the machines lying by the roadside with a "free" sign attached to them? So much for fancy shmancy equipment. On the other hand, if you do like it, then pat yourself on the back and continue because this diet has to please you, not me.

The main point is to make exercise a habit. What's going to make you put down this book and pick up the sneakers? I'll tell you exactly what: it's knowing that exercise lets you can eat more and weigh less forever. You see, exercise moves food through the body at a faster pace, which means that fewer calories will be absorbed. So you could be eating more yet still be losing weight. Exercise also puts you in the fat-burning mode, maintaining muscle while lowering body fat, which translates to looking better.

I understand how exercise can become a habit and even an addiction. However, the opposite can also occur. Once you get out of the routine, it then becomes an effort. Procrastination sneaks into everyone's lives. The key to developing a regular schedule of working out is just to get started. Even if you set aside 10 minutes a day to walk, by the end of the year, that will add up to 60.8 hours of exercise.

I always tell my clients that the best news about exercise is muscle memory. Your body has receptor sites on your muscle strands that are just waiting to be stimulated so they can look sleek and toned. If you've done crunches in the past, your abdominal muscles will show it for months and even years.

The body also secretes endorphins when we train. The body converts them into what we call the "runner's high." Science has proven that those who exercise on a regular basis produce hormones that give them a better outlook and keep them elated and happy!

A dieter must decide that they're willing to exercise. Once your mind is made up, it's time to get the body in motion. Some clients decide that joining a gym is a valuable incentive to continue working out on a regular basis. My advice is to sit down with a pen and paper and write down your five favorite forms of burning calories. Then decide if the things you want to do involve a team, a partner, or if they can be performed solo. Determine how practical each of the activities are in terms of your geographical location. It's obvious that a person who loves to ski won't be doing much of it if they reside in Florida. You should have a varied workout schedule so you don't grow bored of your routine. It's something you have to live with, so why not enjoy it at the same time? Set yourself up for success, not failure! *The first step is to perceive it so that you can achieve it.*

SIMPLE TIPS

1. Start your morning by doing some light housecleaning, such as sweeping, dusting, or doing laundry. This gets the metabolism boosted early in the day, which is the best time to do it, since you have been at rest for several hours.

2. Use the farthest bathroom at work or at home. Every extra step burns calories.

3. Use the stairs instead of the elevator.

4. Walk to close places instead of driving.

5. Park in the farthest spot from your destination.

6. When possible, sit up instead of lying down, and stand instead of sitting. The position of lying down or elevating your legs will reduce your pulse rate and slow down the metabolism. That's why body builders actually gain weight by putting their legs up when relaxing.

A simple thing you can do to offset a modern lifestyle is to walk on a daily basis. As I said, I ask my dieters to just start with a 10-minute brisk walk. The point is to begin an easy exercise program you can live with and fit into your daily schedule. I recently spoke to a woman about how to embark on a diet, and she stated that she was going to walk 5 miles daily because it worked for her once before. I asked her why she stopped doing it if it was so successful for her in the past. She then admitted that she was overwhelmed, and it became too time consuming and physically difficult to do on a daily basis. Then I replied that it really didn't work because it didn't result in permanent weight loss. It just set her up for diet sabotage in the past, so why repeat the mistake? I have been counseling for over two decades, so it wasn't the first time I've heard outrageous exercise plans. I told her that the real reason she does this is that she wants to make the exercise program so brutal that she has an excuse to quit it.

In other words, you can set yourself up for failure in advance. You know in your mind that you can only continue for a short while, so you start with the intention of quitting. Then you tell yourself, your family, and your friends that it's just too difficult to keep up the vigorous exercise program. You stop walking altogether instead of modifying the program so you can get reasonable exercise on a daily basis. If you simply set an achievable goal, you would still be doing something rather than nothing.

If you walk 10 minutes daily, it's 3,650 min. more than you did last year. Once you become accustomed to a regular exercise schedule, it's a natural response to do more as you progress. If you work your way up to 20–30 minutes daily, then you'll be burning even more calories, and boosting your metabolism as an added bonus.

Scientists agree that for every hour of exercise, you add two hours onto your life. I call that a longevity bargain! It's one you can't buy with all the money in the world. All you need to get started is the desire to live a longer and thinner life!

TOP TEN REASONS YOU SHOULD START WALKING!

1. Walking is America's favorite sport. This is because it's the safest way to burn calories and increase physical fitness.

2. Walking is an excellent form of aerobic exercise. It will help strengthen your heart. Scientific studies prove that a stronger heart reduces your risk of heart disease, heart attacks, and high blood pressure.

3. When you walk briskly, your body gets into the fat-burning range, which in turn boosts the metabolism and expedites weight loss.

4. Walking increases energy level throughout the whole day.

5. Walking helps to relieve stress and anxiety.

6. Walking clears your mind and puts you into a better mood.

7. Walking maintains a healthy bone density.

8. Walking helps the body to detoxify via sweating and deep breathing.

9. Walking increases your muscularity, thus allowing you to look better for your weight.

10. Walking works every muscle in your body all at once, and thus promotes overall health and longevity.

EXERCISE FACTS AND FICTION

1. "ONCE I EXERCISE, I'LL BE ABLE TO EAT MORE AND STILL LOSE WEIGHT!"

It's highly possible to gain weight when you exercise with this attitude. Your intent is to lose weight, so focus on the goal, but if you use exercise as a crutch to increase your food intake, you will gain weight. Don't convince yourself that it's okay, because excuses are just a way to condone your overeating.

2. "IF I GAIN WEIGHT WHEN I EXERCISE, THERE'S NO NEED TO WORRY BECAUSE I'M PROBABLY GAINING MUSCLE."

If that were the case, everyone in this country would look like Mr. or Mrs. Olympia. Even though muscle is good, it's difficult for women to gain muscle unless you weight train every day with heavy weights to tear down your muscle. The body repairs the muscle by increasing the size of the individual fibers, and then your muscle becomes larger in size. The average woman is not strong enough to gain muscle. You can give yourself a quick strength test to determine your physical ability. Try to do ten male pushups, if you can't your probably not lifting enough on a bench press to build muscle. The next challenge is the chin-up; if you can't do ten full chin-ups, you're not able to gain much muscle in your back or upper body. The best form of exercise for a dieter is aerobic, because it raises your heart rate and dissipates more calories in less time than any other form of exercise.

3. "I'LL JUST FLATTEN UP MY STOMACH BY DOING SOME SIT-UPS OR CRUNCHES, OR BY USING AN AB MACHINE!"

This is not scientifically feasible, because spot reduction is impossible. In fact, "bodybuilding" includes the word "build" because that's what happens when you isolate a muscle group and perform a weight-lifting movement. When body builders work their bicep, it gets larger, not smaller. They work their abdominals so that the six muscles become larger and can be flexed for the judges. The reason they have a flat stomach is that their body fat is only ten percent, which is one-third the body fat of the average middle-aged woman. If you truly want a flat stomach, the only way is to lose weight and lower your body fat.

It's obviously still a good idea to do crunches, but don't substitute them for a real fat-burning exercise like brisk walking. If you find that the day has passed by rather quickly, and you only have fifteen minutes that particular day to exercise, then take a fast-paced walk. It's important to walk with an upright posture. This is turn will help tone and tighten your stomach at the same time, thus utilizing your exercise time wisely.

4. "EXERCISE MAKES ME HUNGRY."

You think you're hungry when in fact you're unmistakably thirsty. If you observe athletes after a race, the first thing they reach for is water. They even provide water stops at each mile so the runners don't get dehydrated during the race. When you exercise vigorously, it decreases your appetite. I've competed in races at temperatures above ninety degrees, and the only thing I wanted to do when I was done was sit and guzzle some distilled water. When you get done with your workout program, drink pure water until you no longer feel thirsty, and you'll find yourself hydrated and satisfied. You shouldn't let your mind ponder the thought of eating, because your body will turn the thought into an action. You should relax and drink a non-caloric beverage. Once again, remind yourself that weight loss is the goal. A dieter shouldn't use exercise as an excuse to eat!

LABOR SAVING DEVICES

When mankind invented labor-saving devices, it meant that the average person would burn fewer calories on a daily basis. To really put it into proper perspective, you need to take a look at how it affects our daily lives. I will use a day in the life of a diet client named Florence. She wakes up in the morning and presses a button to brew her coffee. In the past, she would have had to fill her coffee pot and stand by while the coffee cooked. Now she pulls out a frozen breakfast and pops it into her *microwave*. In days gone by, Florence would have had to stand by the stove while it cooked, but instead she's already in her shower. Florence gets out her *remote*, opens the garage door, and pulls out her snow blower. In the days of old, she would have gotten out her shovel and used physical labor to clear the snow from her driveway. She even pushes a *button* to warm up her car instead of going outdoors and scraping the snow off. Now she's off to work where she conveniently shuffles into the elevator and is taken to her exact location. In the old days, she would have needed to use the stairs to get to her workplace. She then sits herself down at her desk to retrieve her *e-mail*. In past times she would have walked to the mailbox to get her mail. Florence then sends her messages to the other office via her fax. Years ago she would have had to go to each and every office and deliver the paperwork. She sits in her fancy office chair in a relaxed position, typing into her *computer*. In the past, she would have gathered instructions from her boss and then traveled back and forth between offices to compile her daily information.

It's time for lunch, and Florence takes the *elevator* to the cafeteria where she buys her meal. She's unaware of the calories because the food is prepared restaurant-style. Years ago she would have put together a simple sandwich and perhaps a piece of fruit. Today's special is rather tempting, so she orders a pasta salad primavera with a green salad and dressing. Little does she know that this lunch is at least triple the calories of what she would have brought from home.

She returns to her office and finishes her work. The day seemed stressful, so she decides to order her dinner and pick it up on the way home. In the past she would have arrived home, taken out her pots and pans, and started preparing her meal. Instead, she snuggles up on her couch with her box of *Chinese food* and begins eating. All of a sudden her whole meal is gone within 10 minutes, and the night is still young.

Her favorite program is about to begin, and why not quickly get a dessert before the show starts? After all, she wouldn't want to miss a crucial scene. Now she becomes engrossed in her show and before you know it, the bowl of ice cream is empty. A commercial comes on and she feels like having just a tad more of her favorite snack. As she walks toward the refrigerator, she passes the cookie jar and eats a couple while she's preparing her ice cream.

When the program is over, she takes her dirty plates and quickly tosses them into the *dishwasher*. In the days of old, she would have stood at the sink and washed them by hand.

It's time to get on the Internet and check her email. She sits down in front of the computer and gets snug and relaxed. She decides to surf the net in order to plan her vacation. She contemplates sitting there for a while, so why not have a crunchy snack to munch on while she compares hotel prices? She becomes involved in her vacation plans, and all of a sudden, the whole bag is gone.

It's getting late, so she shuts off her computer and gets into bed to read. When she's finished, she doesn't feel like getting up again, so she *claps* her hands and the lights go out!

All of these labor-saving devices add up to one common denominator: the modern-day dieter burns fewer calories. It's a scientific fact that objects at rest tend to stay at rest. The positive flip side of this law is that objects in motion tend to stay in motion. This means once you start moving, you'll want to continue the behavior. If you simply get up 10 more times each day, and each trip dissipates about 10 calories, you'll have burned 100 calories. This doesn't sound like a lot, but put it into proper perspective and you'll burn 36,500 calories every year. That equates to losing 10-pound in only one year without much effort. The reverse is also true. If you find that you sit more often than you used to, you can gain 10 pounds in one year just by becoming more sedentary.

Labor saving devices	Alternative
Snow blower	Shovel
Weed Killer	Pull weeds by hands
TV remote	Get up and change channel
Dishwasher	Wash dishes by hand
Electric hedge trimmer	Trim shrubbery with hand clippers
Elevator	Walk up the stairs
Light clapper	Get up and turn off light
Automatic car starter	Go out and start the car
Eating out	Make the meal yourself and clean up
Cell Phone	Get up and answer the phone

Think of the true cost of these labor-saving devices!

FITNESS CHART

Listed below is a chart to keep track of each exercise you perform.

LIGHT:

Gardening, walking (2 miles per hour), badminton, stretch exercises, yoga, light dancing.

MODERATE:

Bicycling (5 miles per hour), light aerobics, weight lifting, golf (walking), walking (3 miles per hour), roller-skating.

VIGOROUS:

Swimming, tennis, handball, bicycling (10 miles per hour), skiing, running, walking (4 miles per hour), rowing, jumping rope.

DAY	Type of exercise	Light	Moderate	Vigorous	Total time

19. DIET ENHANCERS

DIETER'S LITTLE HELPER

The diet supplement industry is one of the fastest growing segments of the natural foods business. There's a multitude of options available to a dieter, but the obvious question still remains: "Which diet products really work?" It's a jungle out there, so you need to purchase the supplements that are scientifically proven to work. The ultimate way is to use scientific evidence that provides real data, which isn't tainted or slanted.

After twenty years of painstaking research, I have designed a regimen of diet products that work synergistically to help enhance your weight loss. The first product that a dieter needs is a multivitamin, specifically designed to replace the nutrients that are often depleted because of poor eating habits. The primary reason that dieters experience hunger is that they lack the necessary nutrients to keep their bodies functioning at a healthy level. This program provides ample food volume, and therefore allows you to feel full throughout the entire weight loss process. If you're consuming plenty of low caloric density food and you still experience food cravings, then you need to increase your intake of absorbable high vitamins and minerals. This is easily accomplished by starting my innovative nutrient program. The particular content of each supplement is specifically suited to a dieter's needs. It gives you an edge in order to overcome the changes that you're making in your everyday eating habits. When your body receives the proper nutrients, you'll automatically feel satisfied and experience more energy than you've ever felt before.

The single most common comment that I've received from my customers is: "How do I get as much energy as you have?" The answer was obvious to me, yet it remained a mystery to my clients. This is something I've done every day for over twenty years. It seemed like standard operating procedure to me, yet my clients weren't doing it yet.

The main difference between my clients and myself was the way that we each started our day. When I wake up, the first thing I do is take my supplements. If I have a morning diet consultation and they happen to see me taking all my vitamins, I jokingly reply: "Would you like to share breakfast with me?" Then as I'm taking a handful of nutrients, I tell them that this is what I call the breakfast of champions. I realized that this was what differentiated me, in terms of satisfaction, from the dieters who felt like something was missing. I gave my body exactly what it needed, and it responded by being content. *I tell my dieters that you don't satisfy nutritional deficiencies by consuming excessive calories.* You quell the body's desire for nutrients by replacing what's missing. You could eat all day long, but if you don't receive what your body is longing for, you're still going to feel unsatisfied.

The best way to stave off hunger is to take my multivitamin and multimineral supplement, which has been scientifically formulated to work in conjunction with this diet. These products will naturally enhance your ability to lose weight. It's common sense that once your body is supplied with the nutrients required to sustain good health, the result is a satisfied dieter. This in turn deters hunger and specific food cravings.

The next step on your weight loss journey is to detoxify the liver. The liver is the general of all your organs and acts as a filter to cleanse your blood of undesirable toxins. I compare it to a coffee filter because everyone knows the consequences of reusing their coffee filter. It just doesn't extract the java efficiently, and you end up with a weak cup of joe. This is exactly what happens when you don't clean your liver. You will end up with an organ that doesn't process your nutrients, which in turn leaves your body with a depleted bloodstream.

The benefits of removing the toxins from your liver would be a book in itself. The primary reason that it's beneficial for a dieter to cleanse this important organ is to encourage weight loss. A healthy liver will be able to metabolize fat at a much higher rate than a clogged one. The average American harbors the belief that their liver is fine because it gives them a false sense of security.

If you depend upon the traditional routine laboratory tests performed at your obligatory doctor's appointments, it's time that you're properly informed of the truth about your liver test. If you ask an expert research scientist for the details of the test, they will tell you that by the time an adverse reading shows up, your liver is already 80 percent damaged. It's simply a test that you can't afford to fail. The travesty of the whole issue is that if you wait for the health of your liver, you'll probably need a transplant or a visit to a lawyer to make out your will!

There is a bright side to this story, and the best time to start cleaning your liver is today. There's an herb call milk thistle, that has been shown in scientific studies to repair and rejuvenate the liver. Your main concern as a consumer is to purchase milk thistle extract that is bioavailable with the highest absorption rate. You need not look any further, because the formula that's designed to detoxify and rejuvenate your liver is available for the first time ever to accompany this diet program.

If you're debating whether or not to purchase this product, then it's time to take the quiz listed below. This will show you without a shadow of doubt that every dieter benefits from my liver detoxifier. The questions below pertain to both your past and present, because the damage to this organ is cumulative.

LIVER TEST

	Yes	No
1. Have you ever smoked?		
2. Have you ever drank alcoholic beverages?		
3. Have you ever eaten processed foods?		
4. Have you ever eaten restaurant food?		
5. Have you ever drank tap water?		
6. Have you ever had episodes of overeating?		
7. Have you ever taken prescription drugs?		
8. Have you ever taken over-the-counter drugs?		
9. Have you ever eaten foods with pesticides or insecticides?		
10. Have you ever eaten fried foods?		
11. Have you ever consumed foods with artificial flavors?		
12. Have you ever consumed foods with artificial colors?		
13. Have you ever eaten animal protein?		
14. Have you ever used household cleaners?		
15. Have you ever lived near a main highway or road with consistent traffic?		
16. Have you ever lived near a factory or industrial area?		
17. Have you ever lived near a farm that used chemicals on their crops?		
18. Have you ever exercised on roads where there was motor vehicle exhaust?		
19. Have you ever been employed by a company that produced chemicals?		
20. Have you ever been employed by a company that cleaned with chemicals?		

	Yes	No
21. Have you ever been on a high protein diet?		
22. Have you ever consumed hardened or processed fats? (Such as margarine or vegetable shortening)		
23. Have you ever been constipated?		

After you've taken the liver test, it's obvious that there are numerous dietary and environmental factors that influence the health of this vital organ. If you answered yes to more than three of these questions, then the new liver cleansing formula is a perfect addition to your diet program. This product will enhance your ability to lose weight and increase your metabolism simultaneously. The additional benefit that the dietary supplement called Livafix gives you, is increased absorption of nutrients. When you clean your liver, the supplements that you take will work more efficiently. This in turn decreases your hunger because your body obtains the essential vitamins and minerals it needs in order to stay satisfied.

The next diet helper that's vital to your supplement regimen is Metabofix. This product is specifically designed to replace the nutritional deficiencies that occur when your thyroid gland isn't functioning efficiently. It's a fact that over five million people in the United States have thyroid problems. There are several symptoms that indicate a sluggish metabolism. You can fill out the checklist below to help assess whether your metabolism is slow.

METABOLISM TEST

	Yes	No
1. Do you feel a lack of energy?		
2. Do you have cold hands or feet?		
3. Do you often feel cold?		
4. Do you have a slow heart rate?		
5. Do you gain weight quickly?		
6. Do you lose weight slowly?		
7. Do you experience muscle weakness?		
8. Do you have muscle cramps?		
9. Is your skin dry or scaly?		
10. Is your hair getting thinner?		
11. Do you have hair loss?		
12. Do you suffer from recurrent infections?		
13. Do you have constipation?		

14. Are you sometimes depressed?		
15. Do you ever have difficulty concentrating?		
16. Have you ever suffered from slow speech?		
17. Did you ever have fertility problems?		
18. Have you ever had swollen eyes?		
19. Is your body temperature lower than normal?		
20. Do you ever experience digestion problems?		

Now take a look at the number of yes responses. It's important to note that each question represents a symptom of a slow metabolic rate. This is commonly referred to as hypothyroidism. The condition is caused by an underproduction of the thyroid hormone. Therefore, the more times you answered yes, the more indications exist that your thyroid gland is in need of nutritional assistance.

The good news is that there is a solution to your metabolic problems. The answer to increasing your metabolism is to supply your thyroid with the proper nutrients. Once this is accomplished, your thyroid gland will function more efficiently. When you have a healthy thyroid, your body will produce more thyroid hormones. The increase in thyroid hormones will amplify your metabolism. As a result, you can attain the ultimate goal of every dieter, which is to lose weight quicker and keep it off forever!

The perfect product to boost your metabolism and enhance your weight loss is the Metabofix. It contains a blend of nutrients specifically designed to repair and rejuvenate your metabolism. This product is a perfect addition to your diet program because it speeds up your weight loss. This synergistic blend of nutrients provides you with all the right ingredients for maintaining a healthy thyroid. The specific ingredients and their precise functions are detailed on my website, TheNetCalorieDiet.com or Netcalories.org

Enzymes are the next essential items for increasing your ability to lose weight. They're comprised of long chains of amino acids and are virtually responsible for all of the biochemical activities that go on in the human body. Enzymes are of particular interest to a dieter, because they're necessary for increasing your ability to digest food. The three essential digestive enzymes that amplify weight loss are amylase, protease, and lipase. The function of amylase is to break down carbohydrates. The purpose of protease is to aid in the digestion of protein. The primary role of lipase is to help digest fat. Therefore the quicker you digest your food, the fewer calories your body absorbs. The additional bonus you receive by taking digestive enzymes is that they increase the absorption of nutrients.

The ability to enhance your assimilation of nutrients will in turn help alleviate hunger! The benefits of taking my enzyme supplements are so numerous that there are hundreds of books devoted to the sole purpose of explaining how they enhance your life and promote longevity. The mere fact that enzymes are used to treat over 150 ailments speaks for itself.

Another essential item that qualifies as a dieter's little helper is stevia. It is a safe alternative to consuming artificial sweeteners. The benefits of choosing stevia rather than other types of sweeteners are discussed in detail in the chapter Foods on Trial. When you consider the caloric savings of replacing stevia for sugar, the choice is obvious. The average American consumes 153 pounds of sugar annually, which adds up to 200,406 calories per year, whereas stevia is zero calories. This mere substitution adds up to a potential weight loss of up to 74 pounds per year. Stevia is a versatile sweetener that can be used in baking as well as preparing low-calorie beverages. It can even be used to prepare low-calorie cocktails. After tasting numerous brands of stevia, I decided to market my own product called Sweet Success. This stevia is the best tasting in the industry. It dissolves efficiently and is a wise choice economically. It is a quality product that is unadulterated so that you can savor every moment of your sweet success.

20. FOOD ON TRIAL

FATS ON TRIAL

OPENING STATEMENT:

There is more confusion about fat than ever before. The over-consumption of fat is a direct correlation to the rise in obesity. The United States is now the most overweight country in the world. This in itself makes a statement that we are misinformed consumers when it comes to dieting fads. Diets range from all the fat you can devour to not eating any it all! What's a dieter to do? The first step is to arm yourself with scientific knowledge that comes from a nonpartisan reputable source. One of the most valuable lessons I learned in college was: consider the source! It is important to discern the information you access. There are hundreds of Internet sites to which the FDA sends warning letters and imparts fines because they misrepresent their products. This happens on a daily basis.

One of the first fat misperceptions happened in the early seventies. The food industry had just marketed margarine. Since it was cheaper than butter, it started to appear on kitchen tables everywhere. The public was all of sudden deceived into thinking it was somehow just as good as butter if not better. Some people were even under the assumption that it was lower in calories than butter. The ulterior motive was to save some money and convince yourself that you made the proper choice in order to justify your buying the artificial alternative. Let's take a closer look at the two and expose the truth of the matter. They both contain the same amount of calories and fat.

Butter or margarine: 1 Tbsp. = 100 calories–11 g fat

Now comes the most important chemical difference. Butter is made by churning milk. Margarine is produced by chemists in a laboratory. It is basically hydrogenated oil that is then artificially colored to look like butter. The artificial color can cause cancer, and the hydrogenated fat may lead to heart disease and high cholesterol! Now you understand why margarine costs less than butter. Look at what you are really buying. I nicknamed it yellow lard when I quickly had to describe it to one of my dieters. It's interesting to note that after its invention, the rate of heart disease and obesity increased substantially in the United States.

The second reason the public chose margarine is because the label states that it contains zero grams of cholesterol. This is misleading because it only portrays part of the bigger picture. The way the body absorbs a molecule determines the role it plays in your overall health. Margarine contains hydrogenated and trans fats. Trans fats or trans-fatty acids occur when polyunsaturated fats are altered through hydrogenation. This is done in order to increase shelf life. If a company can keep a product in the grocery store for a longer period of time without it going rancid, they will have a longer duration in which to sell the product. The company therefore reduces their losses due to spoilage and thus increases their profits. The concept was invented to make more money, not for your well-being! The consumption of trans fats raises your cholesterol. They are more harmful than their label indicates because they not only lower your good cholesterol; they also raise your bad cholesterol. Thus setting you up for future diseases such as arteriosclerosis, atherosclerosis, and eventually heart disease.

The main concern of a dieter is to lose weight. It's obvious that over the years you have accumulated an excessive amount of calories that eventually increased the number of fat cells your body contains. Your goal is to reduce your input of calories, increase your output of exercise, and thereby lower your overall body fat. The only way to consume a high volume diet is to decrease your consumption of fats. You can consume 2.25 times the amount of carbohydrates as compared to fats for the same amount of calories. Dieting is not about starvation; it's about conservation. If you choose your calories wisely, you can actually eat more on a diet than when you weren't dieting.

Our next step is to separate the facts from the fiction, or should I say the fat from the fiction.

"THE FIRST FAT I SHALL CALL TO THE STAND IS THE OLIVE."

Diet Court: Could you please state to the jury your full name?

Answer: My proper name is Olea Europea. I am actually the fruit of the Mediterranean Evergreen tree.

Diet Court: How many calories do you contain?

Answer: In my natural state I only have 5 calories per olive. When humankind concentrates and processes me, my calories rise to 120 per tablespoon.

Diet Court: How much fat do you have when you are turned into oil?

Answer: I have 14 gm of fat per tablespoon. Therefore, 100 percent of my calories are derived from fat!

Diet Court: Would you please explain to the jury why your sales have doubled in the last year?

Answer: The industry put out an advertising campaign that promoted the so-called health benefits of my oil.

Diet Court: What type of fat are you considered?

Answer: Olive oil is a monounsaturated fatty acid.

Diet Court: What is the affect of this type of fat on the human body?

Answer: Scientists across the globe have now determined that the positive impact the oil has on cholesterol is relatively modest.

Diet Court: If a person gains weight by adding olive oil to their diet, won't this increase their chance of getting heart disease and an early death from a heart attack?

Answer: Yes, it certainly will.

Diet Court: How much of this type of fat should a person consume?

Answer: The guidelines issued by the National Cholesterol Education Program (NCEP) and widely accepted experts in the field all agree that you should only have 10 percent of your caloric intake come from monounsaturated fats such as olive oil.

Diet Court: That recommendation would only pertain to a healthy, normal weight individual, correct?

Answer: That is true.

Diet Court: How much would a dieter need?

Answer: None, because excess fat and calories only contributes to their weight gain and future health problems caused by their obesity.

"THE NEXT FAT I WILL CALL TO THE STAND IS THE COCONUT."

Diet Court: Could you please state to the jury your full name?

Answer: My proper title is Cocos Nucifera.

Diet Court: How many calories do you contain?

Answer: In my natural state as a fruit and raw, I have 141 calories per half-cup serving. If you dry and shred me, I have 570 calories per half-cup serving. If you pulverize me into a milk form, I am 250 calories per half cup. When you heat and process me into oil, I have 960 calories per half cup!

Diet Court: How much fat does your oil have per half cup?

Answer: I have 112 g of fat!

Diet Court: What percent of this fat is saturated?

Answer: In the oil state, 92 percent of the fat is saturated.

Diet Court: How do you rank amongst other vegetable and animal oils in regard to your percent of saturated fat?

Answer: I have the highest rate of saturated fat. I even contain more of this type of fat than lard, which is 41 percent saturated fat. It is mainly used in the production of cosmetics and soap.

Diet Court: The public has been recently bombarded with an advertising campaign that claims you can help a dieter to boost his/her thyroid function. Would you comment on this please?

Answer: The only thing this oil will do is to boost weight gain. In terms of diet science, let's take a mathematical look at what will happen to an innocent dieter who consumes 4 tablespoons per day of coconut oil. They will be eating 175,200 calories and 19,467 g of fat annually.

Diet Court: What are the consequences of being the oil with the highest saturated fat on the planet?

Answer: The liver uses saturated fats to manufacture cholesterol. Therefore, an excessive dietary intake of this fat will significantly raise your cholesterol level. The most ghastly part of the whole issue is the fact that it raises your bad cholesterol and should be eliminated from your intake in order to lose weight and maintain a healthy lifestyle.

"I WOULD NOW LIKE TO CALL CANOLA OIL TO THE STAND."

Diet Court: Could you please tell the jury your proper name?

Answer: I am actually derived from the rapeseed. I was first synthesized in 1901 by an English chemist name William Normann.

Diet Court: Was this plant initially grown for human consumption?

Answer: No it was not. It was first added to cattle feed to put extra weight on the cows before slaughtering them.

Diet Court: What type of fat are you considered?

Answer: I am a monounsaturated fatty acid.

Diet Court: How many calories do you have?

Answer: I contain 120 calories per tablespoon.

Diet Court: How many gm of fat do you have?

Answer: I have 14 gm of fat per tablespoon.

Diet Court: Therefore 100 percent of your calories are derived from fat!

Answer: That is correct.

Diet Court: Scientists around the world agree that only 10 percent or less of your total caloric intake should be consumed of any type of oil.

Answer: That is exactly true.

"THE FINAL FAT I SHALL CALL TO THE STAND IS THE FLAXSEED."

Diet Court: Could you please state your full name for the jury?

Answer: I am of the Genus Linum, and my proper botanical name is L Usitatissimum.

Diet Court: That's quite a mouthful. Could you please describe what forms you exist as in nature?

Answer: I am the seed of the plant.

Diet Court: How many calories do you contain in that state?

Answer: I have 45 calories per tablespoon

Diet Court: Please tell the jury how much fiber you contain.

Answer: I have three grams of fiber in each tablespoon

Diet Court: This is then considered one of the highest sources of fiber in comparison to other foods?

Answer: Yes, and fiber helps to expedite digestion, which in turn reduces the amount of calories that your body absorbs.

Diet Court: How many calories do you contain when you are ground into flaxseed meal?

Answer: I have forty calories per tablespoon.

Diet Court: How much fiber do you have per tablespoon as flaxseed meal?

Answer: The same amount as my seeds, which is three grams per tablespoon.

Diet Court: What is your calorie count when you are pressed and made into oil?

Answer: The calories are 120 per tablespoon.

Diet Court: Do you retain any fiber?

Answer: No, there is no fiber in my oil.

Diet Court: What differentiates you from the rest of the oils?

Answer: Flaxseed is considered medicinal oil.

Diet Court: Could you please elaborate on what deems you medicinal oil?

Answer: Flaxseed is rich in omega-3 essential fatty acids, and studies have shown it provides many health benefits.

Diet Court: Could you please name the primary ones?

Answer: It is used to strengthen the immune system, lower blood pressure, reduce menopausal symptoms, and lower cholesterol levels. It is essential to solving skin ailments such as eczema or psoriasis. There are books written exclusively on the topic of flaxseed and its medicinal advantages!

Diet Court: How useful is it to a dieter?

Answer: It helps to block the absorption of other harmful fats and in addition reduces the appetite. It also stimulates the fat metabolism at the same time.

Diet Court: How long have flaxseeds been utilized as a food?

Answer: They have been part of the human diet for over five thousand years.

CLOSING STATEMENT:

In closing I would like to state that all fats no matter what type they are contain 120 calories per tablespoon. That's forty calories per teaspoon. While dieting it is important not to waste your calories, even if you think you only use a little bit of oil. A little adds up quickly when you think about all the places it sneaks its way into your diet. If you forget to count only two tablespoons of any oil per day, you will have 240 calories per day totaling 87,600. That adds up to twenty-five pounds of weight you can choose to lose or gain.

I have not had a bottle of oil or any fat such as butter in my home for over 20 years. My clients ask me what I cook with, and I reply "heat!" What they are really asking is what I use to replace oil, and I use water. It has no calories, and it replaces the moisture that the oil would have provided. If I add too much water, it evaporates. If you pour on oil, it remains in the recipe forever and eventually shows up on the scale. The goal of a dieter is to get rid of fat, not look for it!

SWEET REVENGE
(SWEETENERS ON TRIAL)

OPENING STATEMENT:

The search for sweets has been going on for over 2,300 years. In the year 325 BC, Alexander's admiral, Nearchus, wrote about an Indian reed. He described it as a "plant that produces honey, although there are no bees." The man was describing what we commonly refer to as sugar cane. The quest for something sweet spanned the world. Even Columbus was fond of the cane and grew it in Santa Domingo in 1493. As the sugar industry grew, the consumption of it also grew. In the year 1820, Americans ate only ten pounds of sugar per year. Eighty years passed, and by the year 1900, the country was devouring sixty-five pounds per year. The production techniques became more sophisticated, and the product became refined, which meant it was readily available. The consumption increased to 106 pounds per year by 1923. Today Americans gobble up 150 pounds of refined sugar per year!

The confusion of which sweetener to use has been a controversy since the invention of alternative sugars. Each company boasts and brags about the reasons the consumer should choose their particular sweetener. The only way a logical choice can be deduced is by reviewing the scientific facts in order to make the proper decision. It's time to put sweeteners on trial.

"THE FIRST SWEETENER I SHALL CALL TO THE STAND IS SUGAR."

Diet Court: Could you please state your full name?

Answer: My proper title is Saccharum Officinarum. I'm made into several varieties.

Diet Court: Could you please name the most common types of sugar for the jury?

Answer: They are brown molasses, sucanat, turbinado, and white granulated sugar. It's an interesting fact that more than half the world's sugar supply comes from the sugarcane.

Diet Court: Where does the rest of the processed commercial sugar come from?

Answer: The remainder is supplied from sugar beets, which is similar to sugar cane sugar.

Diet Court: How many calories do you have?

Answer: I contain approximately fifty calories per tablespoon.

Diet Court: Do you contain any nutrients?

Answer: No, I contribute nothing to the human diet!

Diet Court: What is your purpose?

Answer: I am used to enhance the flavor of cakes, pies, cookies, chocolate, candy, and other desserts.

Diet Court: Do you have any lasting side effects on the human body?

Answer: Yes, when processed I contribute excess calories to the diet, which leads to diabetes and obesity.

Diet Court: Are there additional problems related to the consumption of sugar?

Answer: Scientists have stated that sugar sets the aging process in motion. It depresses the immune system and causes genetic mutations that can lead to cancer. There are many additional maladies that are caused by eating sugar, so it is best that dieters avoid it or consume it sparingly.

"THE NEXT SWEETENER I SHALL CALL TO THE STAND IS THE GROUP OF SUGARS THAT WE SHALL CALL PLANT-BASED SWEETS. THESE INCLUDE ANY SUGAR DERIVED FROM A PLANT, OTHER THAN CANE SUGAR."

Diet Court: Would you please name the traditional sweeteners in this category?

Answer: They are agave, barley malt, brown rice syrup, date sugar, fructose, and maple syrup.

Diet Court: How many calories do these sweeteners contain?

Answer: They average about fifty calories per tablespoon.

Diet Court: What differentiates them from cane sugar?

Answer: The method of production.

Diet Court: Could you please elaborate on that statement?

Answer: They are taken through less chemical processing steps than processed sugar.

Diet Court: What does this mean to the average dieter?

Answer: The tendency toward addiction is reduced. When you consume sweeteners derived from food, you reduce the risk of health-related disorders. However, they still contribute additional calories to your dietary intake, which in turn causes weight gain.

Diet Court: Are these sweets a better choice than white sugar for a dieter?

Answer: If you absolutely feel a need to eat something sweet, they are a better choice for several reasons. The first and foremost of them is that they are usually used to sweeten natural foods. Therefore, the food doesn't contain artificial flavors. It is a proven fact that the combination of artificial colors and sugar trigger the brain and cause uncontrolled eating. Therefore, a product that contains only natural ingredients does not cause craving in a physical sense. It's important while dieting to choose sweets that don't bring about mental or physical desires to eat them until they are finished. When you consume a natural cookie, you can stop after one or two because they contain whole grains and nutrients that deter hunger.

"THE NEXT GROUP OF SWEETENERS I SHALL CALL TO THE STAND ARE THE ARTIFICIAL TYPES, THOSE THAT HAVE BEEN CHEMICALLY ENHANCED TO PRODUCE A SWEET TASTE."

Diet Court: Could you please state to the jury the most commonly consumed artificial sugars on the market today?

Answer: They are saccharin, aspartame (Nutrasweet, Equal), and sucralose (Splenda). The two most popular sugar substitutes used in America now are aspartame and sucralose.

Diet Court: Would you please tell the jury their actual chemical names?

Answer: Aspartame is L-aspartyl-L-phenylalanine methyl ester. Sucralose is 1,6-dichloro-1,6-dideoxy-beta-D-fructofuranosyl-4-chloro-4-deoxy-alpha-D-galactopyranoside.

Diet Court: That is quite a mouthful. Do these sweeteners have any nutritive value?

Answer: None at all. They are specifically produced to sweeten food and beverages.

Diet Court: Are there side effects associated with aspartame?

Answer: Yes.

Diet Court: Could you please describe some of the most common ill effects of this artificial sweetener?

Answer: The third ingredient in aspartame is methanol.

Diet Court: What does this do to the human body?

Answer: It could be poisonous even when consumed in modest portions.

Diet Court: What happens when you consume toxic levels of methanol?

Answer: The side effects could include blindness, brain swelling, and inflammation of the pancreas and heart muscle. There are so many problems associated with this product that a man named H.J. Roberts wrote a book on it entitled *Aspartame, Is it Safe?*

Diet Court: Could you please summarize the reactions discussed in this text?

Answer: The adverse reactions include headaches, mood swings, changes in vision, nausea, diarrhea, sleep disorders, memory loss, confusion, and even convulsions. The book also points out that aspartame could be dangerous for children.

Diet Court: Just the thought of using it gives me a migraine.

Diet Court: Could you please explain to the jury the recent use of sucralose in the marketplace?

Answer: It was rushed to the food industry due to the onset of the low-carb diet fad. Scientists were pressured to invent a sugar substitute that didn't increase the carbohydrate value of food. In an effort to do so, there is plenty of controversy pertaining to this particular sweetener.

Diet Court: Would you please go into detail for the jury?

Answer: The main concern to the public is its safety. The advertisements lead the consumer to believe that it is naturally derived from sugar.

Diet Court: Are there any safety concerns with this product?

Answer: There are no long-term human studies done to determine the health problems that the sweetener will cause, so avoid this sweetener altogether, since there are other safer alternatives.

"THE NEXT PRODUCT I WILL CALL TO THE STAND IS STEVIA."

Diet Court: Could you please state your full name for the jury?

Answer: My botanical title is Stevia Rebaudiana.

Diet Court: How many calories do you contain?

Answer: None.

Diet Court: Where do you come from?

Answer: I am a small plant that is native to Paraguay and Brazil.

Diet Court: When were you discovered?

Answer: I was recognized by a South American scientist named Antonio Bertoni who learned of the herb from the Guarani Paraguayan Indians. The Indians called it "sweet herb" or "honey leaf."

Diet Court: When was the herb first produced as a sweetener?

Answer: There were two French chemists named Bridel and Laviel who researched the stevia leaves and eventually made them into a white crystalline compound they named "stevioside."

Diet Court: How sweet was stevia?

Answer: The substance is 100 times sweeter than table sugar.

Diet Court: How is Stevia manufactured?

Answer: The non-chemical method of extraction, which was recorded in the herbal manuscripts of Chinese emperors, is still used to this day.

Diet Court: Is this plant considered safe?

Answer: Yes, in fact there are plenty of scientific studies that have shown stevia to be a healthful addition to the human diet.

Diet Court: Is it used in other countries as a sweetener?

Answer: Yes, it is currently used throughout the world in a variety of ways.

Diet Court: Could you please tell the jury what you are considered in the United States?

Answer: I am called a dietary supplement.

Diet Court: Why are you called a supplement?

Answer: The sugar industry has a powerful political impact on this country's laws, and if I divulge any more information, I will be in fear for my life and my industry. I'll have to plead the 5th Amendment on this one!

Diet Court: That's the sweetest supplement you'll ever hear from in your life. Thank you for your information and education.

CLOSING STATEMENT:

In closing, I would like to point out that there are plenty of different sweeteners used by the food industry. You would have to have a degree in chemistry to understand the biological impact these sweeteners have on your health. The simplest way to discern the truth about sweeteners is to review the math. Let's group the sweeteners into two categories. The first of these is the caloric sugars, and the second is the non-caloric sugars.

The sweeteners that contain calories are approximately fifty calories per ounce. The foods that they sweeten are usually cakes, cookies, candy, and other desserts. They are commonly combined with hydrogenated oils and artificial flavors and colors, all of which are known to be harmful to your health. These processed sweets also cause food addictions and chemically affect the brain to crave more of them. Therefore, the more you eat, the more you want. This in turn leads to the consumption of excessive calories, which causes weight gain and ultimately obesity. The goal is to lose weight, so the next time you desire something sweet, reach for a piece of fruit, not a piece of pie.

The non-caloric sugars seem useful to a dieter because they are calorie free. The problem here is they are not free of harmful side effects. You should not consume sweeteners without nutritive value because the body tends to crave the real thing, and you end up eating sweets anyway. Non-caloric sweeteners shouldn't be construed as food because, chemically speaking, they are food additives or substitutes. Why find out twenty years from now that you health problems, all because you chose some high-tech sugar substitute. Plain and simply put, the disadvantages outweigh the advantages—if there were any advantages whatsoever.

It's time that the American public use their buying power to make an impact on the diet industry. It's not logical to support companies that harm your health and contribute to your weight gain. Don't pay for your own obesity! If we choose a dietary supplement (stevia) to sweeten our food, we will be thinner and healthier in the long run.

THE TRUTH ABOUT CHOCOLATE

It took 15 years and a slew of scientists to come up with this ingenious marketing scheme. The ulterior motive was to increase sales of their product. The hidden agenda was to transform the image of this item from an unhealthy one to a healthy one. If the scientists could find even one miniscule reason that would justify the consumption of this food, it would mean billions of dollars worth of additional profits for these companies. The moment the producers were patiently awaiting had finally arrived. A single change in the cell wall was about to transform their product from junk food to a supposed health food. Leave it to a candy company with a larger budget for research than most medical labs to come up with an excuse to eat chocolate! The original statement that was released to the scientific community was that the active components of cacao (theobroma cacao) contain catechins, oligomeric, procyanidins, and flavanoids, which are commonly referred to as antioxidants. The cacao is also a source of theo bromine, which is a mild stimulant. If this sounds like Latin to you, that's because it is. In layman's terms it means the industry would breathe new life into the sales of their dark chocolate. The marketing campaign would shine a ray of light on what was otherwise considered dark (chocolate, that is). It only took moments for the chocolatiers to jump on the bandwagon, or in this case the money-wagon. Then before you even contemplated buying a bar, there were millions of advertisements that told you chocolate is now all of a sudden considered heart-healthy. The truth of the matter is that dark chocolate contains substances similar to heart-healthy compounds in green tea. The key words in this sentence are *similar to*, which in the scientific world means next to nothing because there are compounds occurring in nature that only vary in chemical structure by one molecule. That would by definition of the word make these chemicals similar, yet one could kill you and the other could cause no harm at all!

The point I'm trying to make is simple: advertisements can legally bend and twist the English Language to their advantage in order to sell their products. The whole concept of marketing the so called health benefits of dark chocolate is bizarre because it's as if the media and consumers of the product have forgotten about the calories, fat, sugar, and chemicals in the chocolate. There's no reason to consume excessive calories in order to get antioxidants. As I told my diet clients, when people want to consume a certain food, they will justify eating the item anyway they can think of. There are numerous foods that contain significantly higher amounts of antioxidants than chocolate, yet as one of my diet clients once put it, "But they don't taste as good." Now we're getting to the bottom line of why the consumption of chocolate has tripled in the United States! The scientific fact is that as chocolate consumption soars, obesity and heart disease are also rising and now are at an all-time record high. It doesn't take a genius to figure out that these figures have a direct correlation. It's actually humorous when you think about it because what was once considered a forbidden food is now acceptable to eat in public without feeling guilty. If you really ponder the justification of why we eat a particular food, it becomes clear that people want to feel that what they are consuming is acceptable.

I'll give you some perfect examples that illustrate the acceptable concept. You come home, you find your dieting spouse eating a piece of carrot cake, and they reply, "I'm eating it because it has carrots in it that are packed full of antioxidants." Another case in point is your co-worker brings an apple pie to work and everyone eats it because apples are good for you. This line of reasoning allows you to adulterate a good food and eat the new recipe because it contains one item that has nutrients in it. I suppose that's why the frequent bar patron orders a scotch and water instead of just a shot of scotch because they need their daily requirement of the essential nutrient, water.

Now it's time for a reality check. It shouldn't come as a surprise to anyone that chocolate is high in calories and is not considered a suitable diet food. If you really think about what you're eating when you consume chocolate, you probably wouldn't have taken up the habit of eating it in the first place. The average chocolate bar contains white processed sugar, cocoa butter, artificial colors, artificial flavors, and toxic pesticides.

The reason it maintains texture and doesn't become liquid at room temperature is because of the cocoa butter that it contains. If you want to purchase cocoa butter in a natural food store, you won't find it in the food section because it's not classified as an edible item. The place you'll find cocoa butter is in the H.A.B.A. (Health and Beauty Aids) section of the store, and it's sold as a moisturizer. If you try to look up the calories of cocoa butter in your calorie counter, you won't find it because it's not considered a food! The mere fact that it's a fatty solid chemical at room temperature should provide ample reason that it's unhealthy for you and your heart.

The actual chocolate itself is bitter and therefore requires a sweetener in order to make it palatable. This is typically accomplished by adding processed sugar. There are hundreds of reasons why dieters shouldn't consume processed sugar, but the most obvious one is that it contains chemicals that trigger cravings. It also puts undue stress on the pancreas and leads to diabetes. The chocolate bar contains a dangerous duo that amplifies your level of addiction. It's the dreaded sugar and artificial flavor combination. It leaves the brain wanting more and more, similar to drug addiction. I've asked thousands of clients over the past twenty years, "What food do you find that you can't stop eating once you start consuming it?" The most common answer amongst my dieters is chocolate! That answer alone speaks volumes for itself in regard to uncontrolled eating behavior. Chocolate is a perfect example of a danger food. It's inherent in the name itself that anything that's deemed a danger food should be eliminated from your diet when you're on a weight reduction program. Many dieters do not want to put undue stress upon their dietary discipline by tempting themselves with chocolate. If you're sincerely concerned with getting the active components of dark chocolate, you should take the cacao supplement. Listed below is a synopsis of the consequences of consuming dark chocolate in respect to weight gain and financial burden in a single year.

Dark Chocolate	Cacao
Serving Size: 2 oz.	Serving Size: 2 capsules
Calories: 160	Calories: 0
Calories consumed per day: 160 cal. x 2 oz. = 320 cal.	Calories consumed per day: 0
Calories consumed per year: 320 cal. x 365 days = 116,800 cal	Calories consumed per year: 0
Weight gained per year = 33.37 lbs	Weight gain per year: 0 lbs
Cost per day: $6.25	Cost per day: 15.9 cents
Cost per year: $2,281.25	Cost per year: $58.04

The above illustration should provide ample evidence to eliminate chocolate from your diet. It's comforting to defend your consumption of dark chocolate via the mass media's claim concerning it's so-called "health benefits," but the bottom line is that it's too calorically dense to be part of your daily diet. If you think that a little bit won't hinder your weight loss, then take a good look at what only eating 2 ounces per day will do to your current body weight. This tiny tidbit of chocolate per day could cause a weight gain of 33 pounds by the end of the year, which means it's better not to indulge in order to avoid the bulge!

21. YOUR DIET PERSONALITY

Each person approaches dieting differently, with their own unique attitudes and strategies. It's important to discuss this, because the way you diet will determine your success or failure. This chapter discusses a wide range of diet personalities and how each type can achieve success. The best way to overcome the "dieting syndrome" is to recognize your individual personality and then turn your destructive behavior into constructive behavior!

Let me give you an example. The alarm goes off, and you slowly get out of bed. In the back of your mind you start to formulate diet defense mechanisms before you even begin your program. "It's Monday already, and I won't be able to stop at the coffee shop today, because I know I can't say no to the croissant that I usually have with my cappuccino." You start preparing your children's lunches and you reach for a couple of cookies to put into a baggie and all of a sudden you find yourself, by habit, wanting to pop one into your mouth, but you refrain from doing so. "Ah, my first diet temptation and I overcame it."

Throughout the workday, you continually resist office donuts and other enticements. You finally return home to microwave yourself a diet meal. You know it won't fill you up, but it's quick and it's easy. The meal doesn't take long to eat, and before you know it, the food is gone. Your husband comes into the living room with his evening bowl of ice cream and asks if you want some. "Oh, I forgot you're on a diet, dear. Would you like me to get you a piece of fruit?" At this point you're about to explode, but you quell your emotions and respond with a simple, "Yes, honey, I'll just sit here and eat a peach while you devour your delicious double chocolate almond caramel crunch ice cream." You eat the fruit and decide to retire early, wondering how you will ever make it through another day of dieting!

This may not be your exact case scenario, but you understand that when you diet, your whole life changes. *It's the way you diet that determines your success.* For example, if you take on the "Woe is me" attitude, you eventually feel that you are entitled to binge because you earned it. Your diet personality has a profound effect on your results.

EXTROVERT DIETER

There are personality traits that dieters develop when they embark on a weight loss program. The most common diet personality is the *extrovert dieter.* This is the person who can't wait to tell everyone that they're on a diet. They lose a couple of pounds and they boast and brag to their friends and family of their accomplishment. They start exercising and inform the world of how many inches they have lost off their waist and hips. They are like their own cheerleader. This type of dieter wants the rest of the world to start the diet with them so they can share their good fortune. The drawback with this type of social behavior is that the person goes out on a dietary limb, so to speak. They are on a diet stage, and their family and friends are the audience that sits there and waits for them to perform. If they don't lose weight, they tend to feel like a failure because they have such high expectations for themselves.

The typical profile of an extrovert dieter is a youthful individual who hasn't been on and off diets in the past. It's usually their first diet, and they are eager to lose weight. It's almost as if they discovered a pearl in the clamshell. They tend to go full speed ahead their first week and achieve excellent results. The extrovert dieter even exceeds the expectations of the program. If the diet allows for 1,500 calories, this dieter will consume 1,000 calories just to prove how diligent they can be on a diet. They work out twice as much as the program recommends because this will help them to get to their goal weight in record time.

The extrovert dieter must be aware of their shortcomings in order to obtain their weight loss goal. If you set standards for yourself that are not logically obtainable in the time allotment you prefer, then you don't allow yourself room to succeed. These dieters go above and beyond the call of diet duty in order to achieve immediate results. This is usually done with an ulterior motive in mind. The motive is completion. The dieter starts to think that they can outsmart the system and lose their weight in half the recommended time. Why must the dieter do this? Are they in a "lose more weight quicker than anyone else" contest? The underlying reason is that they want to get the diet over and done with. They usually can't wait to get off their strict starvation plan and go back to their old eating habits. This generally happens after about two weeks, at which point they usually gain all their weight back and more because they celebrate their weight loss by overeating.

How does the extrovert dieter avoid these pitfalls? The key here is to turn your negative behavior into positive behavior. The first thing the dieter must do is follow the program as written. The dietary changes you make must be incremental, not drastic. The energy and passion you have should be used to expand your diet horizons. Since you are an ambitious person, why not channel your talents toward making daily changes that turn a bad habit into a good habit. One way of doing this is to make a new diet recipe once a week so that you become accustomed to cooking low-calorie gourmet meals. If you feel a need to increase your exercise, then take up a new sport. Don't drive your ambition into the ground by doing the same boring exercise day in and day out. Focus on daily changes that you can live with, and incorporate them into your everyday eating habits. Don't put a time limit on your weight loss. Diet one meal at a time, and give yourself some dietary leeway. Remind yourself that you are not in diet boot camp; instead think of it as a diet cruise, and you're treating yourself to all the right foods in order to arrive at your destination—Thinsville!

INTROVERT DIETER

The next diet personality to discuss is the *introvert dieter.* The profile of this type of dieter is a person who has been on and off diets for years. They have been overweight most of their life and don't feel a need to tell the rest of the world that they are on a diet. They tend to keep their dieting a secret. This is done for several reasons, the first of them being the fear of failure. They don't feel like hearing their friends and family make condescending statements like, "Oh, you're trying a new diet," or "How much weight have you lost this time?" The second reason their diet remains confidential is they don't have to adhere to the program in public or in front of their family. If they decide to binge at a party, no one will notice because they aren't aware of the diet. This person usually has a low self-esteem. They feel that others judge them unfairly because they are overweight. They don't want their peers to know that their obesity bothers them. They act as if they accept themselves and don't feel a need to change in order to be socially acceptable. They appear to be happy with their body so that others will not question their eating habits. They don't want to be told what to eat or how to lose weight. They prefer to try a diet incognito, so that when they lose weight, they will show everyone that they really can accomplish their goal in spite of what other people think of them.

The problems that arise from this type of diet personality are due to the way in which this dieter tries to achieve their weight loss goal. First and foremost, the concept of keeping your diet hidden from others speaks for itself. If you really want to change your behavior, why won't you share your desire with your loved ones? You don't have to do this by yourself. As soon as you admit to others your good intentions, they can begin to lend their psychological support. Think of it this way: you are overweight, and you want to be normal weight. That's a fact or you wouldn't be dieting. Now you know that your family and friends are aware of your "weight problem" and would like to help you if you allow them to. If you don't tell them that you're on a diet, they will be thinking, *they really should be trying to lose weight. It looks like they have put on some weight over the years. I wonder what they're doing about the situation.* Everyone can benefit when their peers coach and motivate them toward achieving their goals. Look at how a professional athlete performs once they are part of a team. Every player needs a coach, and every player feels a responsibility to perform when they appear in front of several thousand fans just waiting for them to win. If you want to win the diet game, then utilize your coach as well as your fans!

THE PICTURE PERFECT DIETER

This dieter is the consummate perfectionist. You recognize this person immediately. They are the profile of an obsessive-compulsive personality. When you visit their home, everything is in tiptop shape. They organize their home with precision and even tend to alphabetize their possessions. The perfect dieter will follow the directions of a program with all the best intentions of achieving their weight loss goal.

Let me give you a perfect example of one of my clients who would receive an award, if there were one available, for being the perfect dieter. His name is Doug, and he is employed at a power plant as a computer operator. This tells you that by trade he was trained to follow instructions. I asked him to write down his food intake and consume 1,500 calories per day. I also gave him an exercise chart to fill out each day in order to monitor his progress. He arrived fifteen minutes early for his meeting with all the appropriate paperwork in hand. What he turned in was more like a research scientist's document on a human diet study, and he was the subject of the experiment. The food and beverage chart I gave him was programmed into his computer in 1995, and he had a calorie counting program that would determine his daily caloric intake. He would weigh and measure every morsel of food that he ate with the utmost precision. His exercise chart looked more like the journal of a military man in boot camp. I looked at his paperwork in awe. He used a stair stepper for two hours a day, and as if that wasn't enough, he even gave up his hour lunch break and walked the whole time. My first thought upon reviewing his progress was, "How long can he maintain such a stringent pattern of eating and exercise?" I asked him several questions about his past in order to determine his behavior patterns. He told me he had a sedentary lifestyle and had to battle alcoholism. This speaks volumes about his actions. This type of personality does everything to excess. There are no in-betweens, only extremes. They are the person at the beach who goes running into the water and jumps right in regardless of the depth or temperature of the lake.

This type of dieter usually starts a program with a specific weight loss goal and an exact date by which they want to lose it. This was also true in Doug's case. He was determined to reach his goal weight by his birthday. It appeared that he would do anything in order to lose weight. He was trying his best to be successful in the only way he knew possible. His diet personality was getting in the way of dieting.

Let me explain why this method of dieting is counterproductive to weight loss. The most important reason is because of its limitations. It doesn't allow the dieter to make changes that are incremental. What I mean by this statement is that the dieter doesn't alter their diet; they completely change their whole way of eating. When you make such drastic alterations, it's difficult to adopt them as a way of life. The perfect dieter can't be perfect forever. They are going to break the diet someday, and that's when things get crazy.

When this type of dieter decides to binge, they go all out and eat in a totally opposite manner. They either eat the whole bag of potato chips or have none. They will not eat one cookie; they must consume the entire box. The perfect dieter then becomes the perfect binger. They will not fall somewhere in between because they must do everything to extremes. They falter and begin to eat everything that was "forbidden." This way they are still being perfect, just perfectly bad.

There are several ways that you can overcome this diet personality:

1. Realize that we are all human and thus imperfect. You must face the fact that someday you will eat something that is not on your diet program. At that point, you must stop and think, *I ate one cookie, and now I'm going to forgive myself and perhaps go take a brisk walk around the block and chill out so that I don't continue the action. The walk will help me burn off the additional calories I just consumed, and I'll still be eating less than the whole box.* You need to remind yourself that everyone makes mistakes and move forward, not backward.

2. If you have a bite of cake, you don't have to eat the whole thing just because you want to complete the tasks of eating dessert and leaving a clean plate. At that time, you should walk over to the garbage can and throw the rest away. The food is all gone, and the plate is empty, so you have still completed your duty.

3. If you absolutely feel the compulsion to eat the whole bag of snacks, then purchase a smaller product so you can consume the whole bag and still stay within your daily calorie limit.

4. You must plan in advance for the temptations that will befall you. If you know you are attending a party this weekend, then contemplate each item you will be eating and determine in advance how much of each food you will consume.

5. The best way to overcome your compulsion to either starve or gorge is to stop punishing yourself. Think about it. Whether you are losing weight or gaining weight, it is not pleasurable. Ask yourself what would make you happy in the long run. If you just listen to the instructions of this program instead of trying to alter it in order to expedite your weight loss, you will feel full and satisfied every day. Focus on making small changes in your daily eating habits, and diet one meal at a time.

THE DOOMED DIETER

This particular dieter is one who incorporates failure before flight; they diet expecting not to succeed. They know that they have to lose weight, yet they have already made up their mind that it is impossible for them to reach their weight loss goal.

One client came to me only after her sister joined the diet, and it sounded like a good thing to do together. The doomed dieter didn't make the initial contact or appointment. Her sister called on her behalf. She was quiet during the meetings and seemed to be dieting because her sister was encouraging her to do so. Her name was Sharon, and she was the younger of the two sisters. Her older sister's name was Linda. The influence of an older sibling can have a powerful impact on your life, and all she was trying to do was to help her sister lose weight, so they figured that they would help each other achieve the goal.

Sharon lost weight her first week as all dieters tend to do, and then along came the second week. Linda, the older sister, lost more weight than Sharon, as was expected, because she was the person who initiated the plan in the first place. After about the third week, Sharon stepped on the scale and said, "I don't know why I diet. I am always going to be this way." This sentence alone put her attitude in perspective, and I knew that she was determined to fail. You could have the most perfect diet in the world, and those who don't want to benefit will simply sabotage their weight loss plan in order to quit dieting.

The next step was to determine the reasons she had developed such an attitude. I asked why she felt that being normal weight wasn't within her reach. Sharon told me her tale of woe as follows. "I have had this cellulite on my legs for years, and I'll always have rocking chair arms. I crave sweets on a daily basis, and when I can't have them, I become upset and depressed. How can I ever expect to be normal weight?" I asked, "Why do you feel a need to consume chocolate on a daily basis when you know that it impedes your weight loss goal?" The story unfolded as we spoke. Sharon stated that ever since she was a child her grandparents visited them on weekends and special occasions, and they came bearing sweets and treats for their beloved grandchildren. The sisters would therefore relate their childhood memories of love and affection to the desserts they would enjoy with their family. How this translates to the present day is the process of association. What I mean by association is that when she ate sweets, she felt happy and secure. It is a way to temporarily escape the pressures and stress of life by remembering a time when life was simple and carefree. Then reality hits you, and pangs of guilt seep into your mind. You start to think, *I'm supposed to be on a diet. Why am I doing this?*

There are many reasons why we choose certain foods over other foods, but the plain and simple fact is that everyone has fond recollections of eating comfort food with their loved ones. There are numerous cooking experiences I will cherish for the rest of my life that transpired between my grandmother and myself. I can recall them in my mind (and relive the memory) without ever eating a morsel of my childhood favorites. Since we all have memories attached to food, there has to be a point in your life that you become responsible for maturing from childhood eating habits to eating in an adult manner. If you absolutely cannot reverse the behavior all in one fell swoop, then do it in increments. When you feel the urge to cook an old-time favorite, take the recipe and turn it into a low-calorie version of the dish and have a truly sweet experience, one that lends its way to weight loss and also establishes a new diet personality. The doomed dieter now becomes the determined dieter.

THE "KNOW IT ALL" DIETER

You're familiar with this person because they have quite a diet façade. This is the dieter who's always advising others of the most recent fad diet. They have a carb counter in one hand and a fat counter in the other hand. This person looks at every number imaginable on the label, yet they ignore the most pertinent figure, the calories. They have spent most of their life trying to figure out how to lose weight without counting calories. The problem with this dieter is they really have never faced reality. They have tried to beat the system, and the results are obvious: the system beats them, and they still end up overweight.

I'll give you a perfect example of this type of dieter. Her name is Starr, which is an amazingly appropriate name for her, considering she has played a role in almost every major diet the industry has tried to sell to America. When fat counting was the "in" thing to do, she would stay away from fats, yet it wasn't working because she never really kept track of the number that determines her weight. Then the low-carb fantasy came along, and Starr decided this was the important figure she should pay attention to, but in spite of all her efforts, she still wasn't losing weight. When the facts and figures you pay attention to are only part of your total intake, all you are doing is driving yourself diet crazy.

The strange part about the whole thing is: why concentrate on a number when you don't keep track of the total anyway? If you only count part of your food intake, what happens to the rest of the food that you supposedly left out of the picture? The scale knows and counts every calorie you consume whether you choose to count them or not.

Needless to say, Starr came to her senses after years of trying to avoid the inevitable. She now counts her absorbed calories and is losing weight every week. The important part of counting the correct number is that it always results in weight loss. It has a two-fold advantage in respect to your dietary success. First, it teaches you how to choose between certain foods in order to maintain weight loss. You can now select the lower-calorie foods and enjoy them with the security of knowing you have made the right choice. Secondly, you will not be deceived by unscrupulous labels that lower their carb counts in order to sell to the innocent and ignorant dieters. There are plenty of companies out there with FDA citations and fines because they falsified their carbohydrate counts in order to sell the product.

There are also dieters who that think they need to count sodium in order to lose weight. This just distracts you from the real number, which is calories. The only thing sodium does in reference to weight loss is cause water retention. I'll tell you as a lifelong dieter, I prefer water retention to fat retention. If you consume extra water as a result of the sodium, it actually benefits the dieter because the water and salt helps the dieter feel full. There's nothing wrong with this.

The whole point here is to face the facts that in order to lose weight you must count the only number that results in weight reduction. You could spend your whole life analyzing labels and still end up overweight. The goal here is to lose weight; so the sooner you start counting your net calories, the quicker your scale will start responding.

THE DECEITFUL DIETER

This particular dieter is the most difficult to recognize. They want the rest of the world to think that they are always dieting but just can't seem to lose weight. The person eats all the proper foods in public, yet in private they binge. The problem with this dieter is it's difficult for them to obtain psychological support from their family and friends because they keep their deception to themselves. The person is ashamed of their actions and cannot face themselves, let alone confess their diet sins to others.

I could write a whole book about different clients that fit this personality because it is more common than the public thinks. Let's use a family example to show how peer pressure affects one's desire to lose weight.

We enter the world of the Jones family. The daughter, Jennifer, joined the program first, and after her family saw her lose weight, they were curious. She lost enough weight to start dating, and as fate would have it, Jennifer found the love of her life and got married. This is a perfect example of what successful weight loss can do for your life.

Jennifer was so excited about her new life that she advised her father, Keith, to join the diet. He came to me as a determined dieter and lost over thirty pounds. At this point, he told me that his wife, Carol, would be coming to the diet program. He made an appointment for her, and she arrived in my office the next week for her first meeting.

I prepare mentally for each diet client, and I felt confident that I would be able to help my client's wife. Since her husband was already losing weight, it's a logical conclusion that when a spouse joins, they will be working together toward one common goal: weight loss.

Carol came to my office, and after one glimpse, I was fully aware of the fact that she needed to lose at least 200 pounds. These cases are challenging because the client knows they need to diet for at least a year in order to even approach their goal weight. I had her weigh in, and I measured her. She was shy and introverted as a result of her obesity. Carol was hiding behind her weight, so to speak. We started to chat, and I asked her why she decided to join the diet. She casually replied, "If I don't lose weight, my husband will divorce me!" The thought swirled about my mind, *Oh, not that nice gentleman Keith who has already lost over thirty pounds on my diet. I can't imagine he would do such a thing.* Then I replied to her that since Keith was serious, we'd better get started.

When your motive to diet is not fueled by your own initiative, things don't always work out the way you plan. She didn't exactly want to diet; she was forced to diet or lose her husband. This seems like a rather drastic measure to take in order to get your wife to lose weight, but needless to say, it wasn't the first case, and it won't be the last.

Carol seemed so desperate that I was determined to do everything in my power to help her lose weight. The only thing I couldn't do was diet for her; that part was something she would have to do. She came back the next week and lost five pounds and five and one-quarter inches, yet there was something wrong. You can call it my diet sixth sense, but I knew there was more to this than met the eye. Carol didn't seem happy when she lost weight, which is highly unusual for a second week dieter.

I ask each dieter to write down what they consume and count their calories on a daily basis. They turn in their journal to me, and I use it as a learning tool to help them make dietary changes that will result in weight loss. When asked for her food and beverage recording chart, she handed me a chart with writing on only two of the seven days. Carol was only willing to write down what she ate for two days of her life, and yet she still lost five and one half pounds. I would be ecstatic, yet she didn't seem thrilled. She didn't even add up one single calorie on those two days. All she did was keep a record of what she ate.

Carol lost weight for the next three weeks without completing her diet journal. I would review what she ate verbally, and she seemed hesitant to discuss the details of her food consumption. On the fourth week, she called to postpone her diet meeting. Carol did not come to her appointment for twenty-one days. On the twenty-second day, she came to her meeting, and she stepped on the scale for the first time in three weeks. I knew she was skipping her diet meetings for a reason, and it's usually because the client is on what I deem "diet vacation." This wasn't just a vacation; it was more like a three-week binge session, because she had gained twenty-four pounds in twenty-one days!

It was a miracle in itself that she came back to the diet. Carol was shocked when she stepped on the scale, and she had the look of despair in her eyes. I advised her to look to the future and step forward, not backward. Each day the sun comes up to give us a fresh start in life, and that is how you should view your diet progress. Now Carol was determined to lose the weight she had gained and was a woman on a mission. Carol scheduled her diet meeting for the next week and left after receiving her pep talk.

In the meantime, her husband, Keith, came for his diet meeting. He was losing weight as usual, and all of a sudden Keith shifted the conversation over to his wife, Carol. He told me that he suspected her of eating behind his back. I asked him why he would presume such a thing, and he stated that she had done this before. Keith decided to act upon his suspicions by investigating the supposed crime scene. Keith predicted Carol was binging in her vehicle while traveling to and from her workplace. He offered to clean the car, and his doubts were confirmed. In the trunk was a bag well hidden from sight that contained numerous packages of fast-food meals Carol had eaten in her car. I then asked him if he had confronted Carol. Keith said that he was so upset that he didn't want to discuss it with her because he felt the situation would spiral into a major battle. Keith asked me to take care of the matter instead.

Carol then showed up for her diet meeting and had such a fantastic week that she lost seventeen pounds in only six days! It's common for dieters to try to make up for weight gain with rapid weight loss. This is their form of diet punishment. Now she felt back in control of her diet and scheduled next week's appointment. Carol had such a phenomenal diet week that I decided not to discuss her fast-food binges. Perhaps she would conquer her private eating episodes as a result of her current weight loss accomplishment.

The next week she came to her appointment and had lost two pounds, but again she hadn't written down her food intake. I then asked her to give me a synopsis of her diet, and she told me the details she had kept secret for a long time. Carol admitted eating behind her husband's and two daughters' backs. She was embarrassed and distraught. Carol was using food as a crutch and couldn't seem to break herself free from the chains of obesity. She had such a low level of self-esteem that she let food become her way of nurturing herself. The guilt she felt became overwhelming, and she needed to discuss the situation in order to make sense of her actions. I told her there were two options, and she had to be the one to make the choice.

Option 1: Since you choose to eat in private and can't seem to stop the activity cold turkey, then eat fewer calories in private. If you decide to stop at a fast-food restaurant on the way home to binge, then choose the lower-calorie menu items. If you can't stop yourself, then have a hamburger, subtract the fries, and order a diet soda. If you decide to sneak some cookies in your car, then buy a single-serving package out of a vending machine. If you reduce your solitude calories, you will be taking a step toward dieting.

Option 2: Face the fact that you are not really dieting. If you only reduce calories when in public or in front of family and friends, then you are putting on a show instead of changing your eating habits. It's up to each individual whether he or she chooses to fess up and divulge their secret eating binges. If you aren't ready to tell it all, then keep a private diet journal and add up the calories of your deceitful dieting episodes. Now you understand why you are not losing weight or your weight loss is at a standstill. If you eat calories behind other people's backs, just remember you can't hide the calorie from the scale. It always knows how much you have eaten. You are only fooling yourself and your loved ones. If you continuously tell others you are on a diet and don't lose weight, your actions will speak louder than words. After the years go by and you are still overweight, the world will take less merit in your diet endeavors!

THE MIDNIGHT MUNCHER

This is the dieter who awakes in the wee hours of the night and decides that they are in the mood for a middle of the night snack. It's more common than you would think. The reason is that most dieters don't divulge their binges to the public. The profile of a midnight muncher is similar to the deceitful dieter in respect to the fact that they both eat in private. They also both consume calories without admitting their habits to their family and friends. Some, however, eventually are caught in the act because a family member happens to wake up and discovers their loved one with their hand in the cookie jar .Let me give you a perfect example of this type of dieter.

Her name is Maryann. She came to me with a specific goal in mind. Maryann wanted to lose weight and run a marathon. She worked at a bank and was an organized individual. I expected that she would excel on this type of program because she seemed like a disciplined person. I gave Maryann her diet instructions for the week, and she was exuberant at the prospect of losing weight. She came to her second diet meeting with all the appropriate paperwork and all the pertinent facts and figures. Maryann wrote down what she ate every day and counted her absorbed calories as she was instructed to do for her diet. She lost two pounds and two and one half inches her first week, which is just about perfect for her body weight and food intake. Maryann seemed like a diet counselor's dream come true, a truly dedicated dieter. The kind they write testimonials about and use to sell their program. After twenty years of giving diet meetings, I don't get overly excited without positive proof that the client is really on the diet program. It's a fact that plenty of people can diet for one to two weeks. The real test comes after the diet infatuation stage.

This is similar to your first date. It's the time when you put on your best behavior in order to make a good first impression. Everyone who starts a diet does so with the thought in mind that they will lose weight and end up thinner than when they started the program. The topic is explained in detail in the section of your diet personality entitled The Rookie Dieter.

Maryann came back for her second week and gained three quarters of a pound. She wrote down her food intake and everything looked to be in tiptop shape except for the number on the scale. She then admitted to me that she might have forgotten one or two items that she consumed in the middle of the night. My suspicions were well warranted because the calories she said she consumed would normally result in weight loss. In order to fully comprehend the situation, let's take a look at the underlying factors. Maryann was living with her in-laws at the time because her father-in-law and husband were busy building their new dream home. They were a newly married couple at the time, and I felt that they were being deprived of their newlywed privacy. This was putting a strain on the marriage, and the results were taking their toll on her dieting program. Maryann felt trapped in her situation, and she would escape by eating alone in the wee hours of the night when no one could judge her or discover her secret eating habits.

Maryann told everyone at the bank she was on the program, so she didn't dare binge in front of her co-workers. Her diet personality wouldn't allow her to expose any diet weakness in public. She also told her husband and in-laws about her diet and therefore felt that she couldn't let them down by seeing her falter, let alone fail at her weight loss goal. Maryann was such a determined person that she didn't allow the rest of the world to view her mishaps or binges. She felt that she could make up for her late night eating by exercising. This doesn't work because you tend to consume far more calories than you can burn by working out. She then joined a running club and proceeded to work toward her athletic goal, which was to compete in a marathon. The third week she lost weight, which is common with this type of personality. They tend to punish themselves for their weight gain by losing more weight than they gained. Now she felt back in control of the situation and on the road to achieving her weight loss goal.

The weeks passed by, and I began to see a strange pattern. Every time Maryann had a fantastic week, she would gain weight the next week. I decided to discuss the problem and uncover her diet secret once and for all. Once Maryann admitted the truth, she could then take action in order to change her behavior. I asked her if she slept through the night, and Maryann replied that she didn't feel comfortable at her in-laws house, so she usually ended up getting up in the middle of the night to go to the bathroom, and you have to go past the kitchen in order to get to the bathroom. Maryann finally admitted that she would go to the cupboard and start eating peanut butter from the jar. That was rather dry, so she took out a container of chocolate frosting and started eating the two together. All of a sudden she realized the containers were both empty, and she couldn't face the reality of breaking her diet, so she discarded the bottles in the bottom of the trash so that they would be out of view and went back to bed. The next morning she acted as if nothing happened, and now Maryann had to figure out how to negate these excessive calories. If Maryann wrote them down in her diet journal, she would be over her daily caloric intake. Maryann couldn't acknowledge the fact that she would break her diet. I was the only other human being on earth who knew her secret, and now the ball was in my court. I knew I would be able to solve her problem if she would listen to my instructions. One of my most successful dieters put it into a simple statement. She told her friend, "Go to the diet and do what Donna says, and you'll lose weight!" Advice is much easier to give than it is to follow.

I told Maryann that her stay at the in-laws' home was only temporary and that this was a time burdened behavior. What I mean by this is that her actions were a result of her change in environment. She was reaching for comfort in a home that wasn't hers. If you overeat food because you are in an uncomfortable environment, then there are two options available in order to change or alter the habit. The first is the most obvious: you need to change your surroundings. Ask yourself if it's worth the consequences.

Are you willing to be overweight in order to compensate for your current living conditions? If it's within your reach to change your circumstances, then by all means do so. If you can't alter your external conditions, then change the food you eat in the middle of the night. In my client Maryann's case, I instructed her to eat a low-calorie version of peanut butter, and instead of dipping it into frosting, I told her to put it on an apple or a rice cake. You have to understand that calories are absorbed whether you eat them in public or in private.

The other option is to prepare for the behavior in advance. If you know that you have a tendency to get up in the middle of the night, then drink less fluid after dinner. This will reduce the urge to get up and go to the bathroom, thereby avoiding the kitchen, which tends to prompt the action. You can also try some calming herbs, tinctures, or supplements to help ensure a sound night's sleep. It's completely up to you to make the decision to eat or not to eat. Remember, you control the food, it doesn't control you. You should give yourself time to adjust your behavior. If you really need to get up at night, do yourself a favor and fill a large glass with ice cubes and water. It's zero calories, and you're probably thirsty, not hungry, from the food intake that day.

It's a known fact that diet foods tend to contain more sodium in order to make up for the reduction of fat and calories. You can easily mistake hunger for thirst because the brain doesn't have an independent sensory neuron between the two thoughts. The best plan of action is to drink some pure water and return to dreamland!

THE ROOKIE DIETER

The title seems to be an obvious description of this particular dieter, yet it doesn't tell the whole story. When a person embarks upon a diet, you would say that they are a rookie or virgin dieter because it is the first time in their life that they are dieting. Millions of Americans each day claim to be on a diet, yet they aren't counting their calories. If they don't know how much they consume on a daily basis, then they are not on a diet.

I'll give you a perfect example of this type of diet personality. The person called me up on the phone as a referral. These are usually exuberant and excited individuals because they are anxious to lose weight just like their friend that told them about my program. The client's name was Susan. Her friend, Delores, had lost over 20 pounds on the program and even maintained her goal weight, so Susan wanted a piece of the action. She came with a long history of supposed dieting. Susan had tried pills, shakes, exercise equipment, and starvation and was reading all the appropriate magazines and articles that promise speedy weight loss. I asked her one pertinent question. Have you ever written down what you have eaten for one day and then added up your total calories for that day? She replied with a prompt no. I then told her that the good news is that you have never been on a real diet and you therefore are a rookie dieter. This is a new beginning, I explained, and you now can have a fresh start at losing weight. I instructed Susan to forget all the past experiences she had with trying to lose weight and consider this day to be the first day on her new diet. Susan was elated to finally hear the truth. If you truly want to lose weight, then you must be responsible for what you eat on a daily basis. Susan lost 5 pounds and 6 inches in only one week.

She was surprised when she stepped on the scale because Susan complained that no matter what diet she was on, she never lost weight. I had to reinforce the point that she had never been on a weight loss program. These were just fad diets and gimmicks that lure you into false weight loss promises. Don't let past performance determine your future accomplishments. It's important to learn from the past, perform your best at the present time, and plan and anticipate your goals and dreams for the future! Susan left her past behind her, where it belonged, and by the end of only 30 days, she lost 12 pounds and 15 inches. A real diet really works! So, prepare yourself for success and start this program, knowing that you will never need another diet again!

THE SPECIAL OCCASION DIETER

This type of diet affects everyone at some point in life. It's time to go on a diet because we have to go out into the public, and we're concerned about our social appearance. It commonly occurs when have a wedding, high school, or college reunion to attend. It also happens prior to going away on a vacation because the dieter usually cavorts to a warm environment and as a result wears more revealing attire than their normal wardrobe. The problem with the diet personality is that you are trying to lose weight in order to please others, or in some circumstances, the motive for the weight loss is to impress other people. Either way the point is that you're not dieting for yourself. I asked plenty of clients why they try so hard to lose weight for a group of strangers on a cruise ship that don't even know their name? The flip side of this type of dieting is that it's great news that you've decided to lose weight, and if the event provided a reason to go on a diet, then bravo!

The next step is to put you into the proper diet frame of mind. The reason you went on the diet and you're losing weight is because the social event gave you a sense of urgency. You should take this diet enthusiasm and use it to your advantage. Don't set unrealistic weight loss goals only to find yourself so depressed about not losing the exact amount of weight you desire that you quit dieting altogether. You need to allow yourself time to change your eating habits so that weight maintenance becomes a way of life instead of a quick two week fixer up diet.

This diet personality can get in the way of the best laid diet plans because once the important event approaches and passes, so does the diet. What I mean by this is when the event happens you feel that you have earned the right to go off the diet and eat anything you want to. This often results in a binge that lasts for the duration of the event. If for instance you diet prior to your two-week cruise, the first thing a dieter wants to do is get on board and celebrate. They then do so by consuming excessive calories for the entire two-week vacation. This generally results in weight gain and guilt. It's an unfortunate fact that most dieters end up weighing more than when they started their special occasion diet. This usually leads to an extended period of overeating and more weight gain.

There is a solution for this diet personality. The single most important thing you need to do is to continue the diet with a renewed state of mind. You started a diet to impress others. It wasn't necessarily the right motive, but it got you started. So now you are losing weight, and the event is approaching. Now it's the time to think about your situation. You have already proven to yourself that, when you want to, you can lose weight. That's a fact! So use your past performance in order to provide stimulus to achieve your weight loss goal. It's time to ask yourself why you really want to lose weight. If it's because you are self-conscious about your appearance in front of strangers and acquaintances, then what about your friends and family? Don't you want to feel good about yourself in front of the people you live with and work with? Now take out a pen and paper and write down the top ten reasons you want to reach your goal weight. You should think about the bonuses that come along with losing weight. Your health problems will be lessened and in most cases completely alleviated. When you lose weight, you live a longer and happier life. It's time to make every day a special occasion and diet for the long term, not just a quick fix.

THE SEASONAL DIETER

In the Northeast, it happens after the winter thaw and a cold and dreary spring has passed. It's the first warm day in May, and my phone starts to ring. There's a desperate individual on the other end who needs to make a diet appointment as soon as possible. Their goal is to lose that winter weight gain by summer time. They realize that when they try on their warm weather attire, their clothes either don't fit, or they don't like the way their body looks in those shorts, and the bathing suit is much too revealing at their present body weight. It's time to get serious and lose weight. What the dieter fails to think about is the time factor that's involved. If it's May 15th, and summer starts on June 21st, that only gives the dieter 5 weeks to lose weight before the season starts. If you lose 2 pounds per week, that's a total of 10 pounds. If you have more weight than that to lose, then you shouldn't set unrealistic weight loss goals. This only results in a disgruntled dieter who starts to think, *why bother trying to get thin by summer!* The point here is that you should keep dieting long enough for it to succeed. You know you won't really enjoy the summer when you're ashamed or embarrassed about the way you look, especially when you have to put on a pair of shorts and sit there feeling uncomfortable at the company and family cookouts!

It's time to think about your past dieting performance. How many summers have you done this to yourself? If you had just stuck it out and stayed on the program, you wouldn't be so discouraged right now! This is not your last summer, so don't put yourself in a situation that results in you feeling the same way next summer. It's time to stop putting time limitations on your ability to lose weight. The days pass you by anyway, so why not diet instead of letting the season depart and stay the same weight or in some instances gain weight!

The warm weather is a perfect time to lose weight because you can burn extra calories doing outdoor activities. I look forward to mowing my lawn, clipping my shrubbery by hand, and planting my seedlings in my garden on my hands and knees and working the soil with only a small spade so that I get a better workout. These activities allow me to burn more calories and boost my metabolism at the same time. It's time to take advantage of the summer season instead of it taking advantage of you.

The summertime is an excellent season to experiment with refreshing and nutritious salads. It's the time when produce is at its peak and tastes better than you ever imagined. You should prepare new low-calorie versions of your favorites and enjoy them without guilt or weight gain. Refer to the recipe section for simple yet exquisite versions of pasta and potato salads. You should try a different or exotic fruit or vegetable each week in order to satisfy as well as entertain your appetite. It's time to use your imagination and enjoy the abundance of fresh fruits and vegetables in low-calorie recipes. You shouldn't feel guilty for eating; instead, you should feel nourished and blessed by trying some wholesome organic food that is waiting to tantalize your taste buds.

THE WEEKDAY DIETER

This is perhaps the most common diet personality in America. The Monday through Friday schedule is how we structure our lives. As a culture we are in the habit of starting diets on Monday. After all, it's the beginning of the school week/workweek, and our life is more ordered during that particular time. This sounds like a logical plan of action; however, it presents several pitfalls for the dieter. It all starts out with good intentions on Monday. This is the day that people eat the least amount of calories and adhere to their diet with more diligence than any other day of the week. It's a fact that plenty of dieters know in advance that they will go off their diet on the weekend and celebrate by overeating. The thought in the back of your mind is this: *I've been dieting all week, so what's the harm in forgetting about my diet for two days? It's only the weekend, and after all, everyone else is partying and going out to dinner, so why can't I? I'll go right back on my diet on Monday, but until then I'm going to eat what I want and have a good time. I deserve it because I've had a stressful workweek, and I don't want to ruin my weekend by dieting.*

This line of reasoning will sabotage your diet, because pure mathematics will always win! Suppose you eat 1,200 calories a day for 5 days, and then on the weekend, you consume 2,500 calories per day. That's a weekly total of 11,000 calories, or an average of 1,571. You were supposed to have 1,200 calories per day, but your weekend binges raised your daily average to over 1,500. That may be the difference of losing weight or gaining weight. Therefore, it's important to calculate your weekly *average* calories in order to promote weight loss.

Let me point out that in the above example the dieter stuck to the program on Friday. This is generally not the case because Friday is a payday for most Americans, and it kicks off the beginning of the weekend. This generally means eating out and having a couple of cocktails, which usually puts the dieter well over their caloric intake for that day. If you look at the situation, realistically how may dieters adhere to their program on Friday nights? If you want proof, take a drive past a restaurant or tavern on Friday evening and look at the parking lot. It's usually full, and the patrons are not inside eating a green salad with diet dressing. They are there to eat, and they want their money's worth!

Since most dieters tend to consume more calories on the weekend, which starts on Friday, it really boils down to only dieting four days a week. The most important aspect of this diet personality is that it doesn't promote consistency and often results in weight loss followed by weight gain. If you lose three pounds by the end of the week and gain it all back during the weekend, then you're right back to where you started, which of course is not your goal. You are on a diet to lose weight and adopt eating habits that result in permanent weight loss. If you have been a weekday dieter for an extended period of time, just ask yourself one question. Do you weigh less than you did last year? If the answer is no, then this type of dieting is not working for you; it's only frustrating you.

There are solutions for those dieters who absolutely feel a need to consume extra calories on the weekend. It's a weekend, and you have some spare time on your hands, so utilize it by doing some additional exercise or participating in a sport. This way you burn additional calories and hopefully offset the consumption of an increased food intake. You can also consume 200 fewer calories on Wednesday and Thursday, and then you can utilize your saved calories on the weekend. The other option is to prepare some of your favorite weekend treats with a new twist, by making them lower in calories so that you can still enjoy your weekend without weight gain!

THE DUTIFUL DIETER

This type of diet personality is quite obvious at social events and restaurants. This is the person who feels a need to finish all the food on their plate. They are typically raised in a family that instills a sense of responsibility toward consuming everything they are served. They encourage you to eat every morsel of food you have been given because it's your duty. They view eating as a project that needs to be completed. It's like waxing only half the floor or dusting only part of the bookshelf and feeling like your work isn't finished until all the cleaning is done. The parents of dutiful dieters often use guilt as a motive to eat every morsel of food you are offered. Their most common form of this guilt was the era where parents requested their youngsters to eat everything on their dish because there were starving children in other countries. This never made logical sense to me, and it was used as a ploy to get me to eat more food than I wanted to. I simply rebutted the excuse by stating that I should therefore eat less so that there would be more food to share with the rest of the world.

The dutiful dieter has this rule ingrained in their mind and feels guilty if they don't eat what is served to them. My diet clients even admit that they will eat food they don't like because it shouldn't be wasted. That is simply not the case, because the food was already bought and paid for, so overeating at this point won't save you a dime. When you do this, it's just a justification for your actions. I asked one of my diet clients why he didn't just discard the food instead of turning himself into a garbage can. Since the food is already purchased and you're not going to get your money back, don't let it cause weight gain.

There is an obvious solution to this dilemma. The dutiful dieter needs to serve themselves. Then the portion sizes and food choices are decided by the dieter, not the host or hostess. If you are at a restaurant and the portion that you order contains more calories than you should be eating, ask the waitress to take it away or pack it up and give the rest of the food to a non-dieter, or put it in your bird feeder. Another pitfall that plagues the dutiful dieter is the practice of eating what other people serve them because they don't want to insult the chef. The chef doesn't have to live in my body, nor does the cook have to weigh in and see herself gain weight.

THE TRAVELING DIETER

This diet personality is one that stems from profession. It happens as a result of eating on the road. The eating habits vary according to income. They range from the typical door-to-door salesperson that barely makes a living and tends to quell his hunger at the local fast-food restaurant, to an executive sales rep. that wines and dines his client at four-star restaurants. The restaurants may vary, but they all have the same outcome, which is weight gain.

Let's take a road trip with a gentleman who works as a traveling vitamin sales rep. and has been one for many years. His name is Andrew, and he was kind enough to share his story and his dieting dilemma. He has been traveling for years, and the restaurant calories eventually caught up with him and caused a 40-pound weight gain. In order to fully understand his present situation, we need to discern the events that led to his current body weight. Andrew doesn't like to eat alone, which is a common complaint amongst my weight loss clients. I ask them if overeating feels like a replacement for having a loved one across the table from them, and they often reply that it doesn't replace the loneliness; it just helps them to forget about it for a while. In Andrew's case, he found a way to replace eating alone by having dinner with a book. He stated that he would not settle down to eat dinner unless he had something to read. I told him I approve as long as he reads this diet book while dining. All joking aside, when you take a closer look as to the ulterior motive behind your food habits and choices, then you will solve your dietary problems.

Andrew provided himself with justification for eating at restaurants. His first reason was he felt that it was a better choice than his other options. He stated that he could be going to a strip bar and drinking or doing drugs, which he considered immoral choices and therefore felt that he established just cause for simply having a restaurant meal. The second excuse he used in his defense was the fact that since the company paid for his dinner expenses, why not enjoy a free meal? It's difficult for salespeople to pass up part of their company perks. There are very few people in the world that can pass up free food. It's a temptation that's difficult to overcome. The pure and simple fact is that we all make the choices we do in life for a specific reason. Every person has an excuse for their actions.

If you decide in advance that your profession is the reason for your obesity, then you have premeditated your own destiny. You made a conscious decision to let your circumstances overcome your desire to lose weight. It's up to you to prioritize your goals. You should decide if you want to lose weight or sit around and use your lifestyle choices as an excuse why you are overweight. Once you make up your mind that your diet is an important part of your life, then you can move forward and make the appropriate changes that lead to weight loss.

There are several options available to the traveling dieter. The first thing you should do is map out your eating path just like you do your trip. If you know that you'll have to stop in a town that has only fast-food restaurants and a diner, then bring your food along and have a quiet meal in the hotel room. The next morning you'll wake up thinner and happier, knowing you made the right food choices. You should call ahead and ask the local restaurants if they have low-calorie menu items available for you to choose from.

It's always advisable to bring along low-calorie salad dressing. The best diet intentions are sabotaged when you pour regular salad dressing over innocent low-calorie vegetables. If you find yourself pressed for time, you can always stop at a supermarket and get yourself a salad on the way back to the hotel. See Dieter's Guide to Dining Out guidelines on how to adhere to your diet while eating out.

The other important factor in dieting is to boost your metabolism in order to burn more calories, in case you end up consuming more food than you anticipated. This can be accomplished by taking a walk either before or after dinner. You should also check into a hotel that provides a workout center so that you can exercise each evening (or morning). This allows you to socialize with other travelers and keeps you away from the lonely hotel room. I've heard plenty of stories about the traveler who ends up sitting in front of the hotel television with a beverage in one hand and a bag of snacks in the other just because they are homesick or bored. There is a simple solution for both of these excuses; if you miss loved ones, then pick up the phone and tell them so and talk instead of eat. If you're bored, then take a walk, visit a local museum, or do some site seeing. Another option is to go to a local gift shop and buy a present for your family or friends whom you yearn to see.

THE VICTORIOUS DIETER
UPDATE OF TRAVELING DIETER

Andrew, the traveling vitamin salesperson, has decided to make a career change in order to stay at home with his wife and child. Andrew called to say he had lost 41 pounds and was very excited to tell his story. The first factor that contributed to Andy's weight loss was the mere fact that staying at home meant he was not eating at restaurants. When you eat out on a regular basis, you're always guessing your calories. I joked with him one day and said it's those mystery calories that eventually catch up with you when you eat at restaurants. When my clients prepare their meals at home, they can accurately determine the caloric content of the meal, which means they're in control of the calories. When Andy stopped eating out on a daily basis, he lost weight immediately.

The second determinant in his dieting success was his reduction of wasted calories. In Andrew's particular case, he was consuming far too many liquid calories. Andy stopped drinking milk and soda and replaced them with pure water. The first thing he noticed was that he felt more energy because now his body was being hydrated with water instead of being dehydrated with soda. The weight loss and renewed virility sparked Andy to exercise, which was the third constituent of his weight loss success. The transformation from couch potato to competing athlete was phenomenal!

It's always enlightening to discern the fuel that sparks the burning desire to get up and start exercising. In Andy's case, the accelerant was to facilitate his weight loss. One of the bonuses that comes with weight loss is that it motivates you to exercise because the two are synergistic. It's encouraging to know first-hand that the ability to change is inherent in everyone. The manner in which you proceed has to speak into your life in a profound way.

The first day Andy started to run, he said that his goal was to just make it to the next corner. Then he practiced running and walking in order to build his endurance. Then before you know it, Andy was in his car clocking a three-mile route. He paced himself within his own physical abilities. This is of utmost importance while dieting because those who set lofty, unachievable goals often defeat themselves, not the program. The days passed, and Andy made good use of each one of them by trying to run just a little farther each time he felt he could. Then all of a sudden, last Sunday while standing on the starting line of a race I was competing in, I heard a kind, familiar voice call out my name. It was Andy, and he was standing there in his athletic attire ready to run the race. I was so happy for him that words wouldn't do my emotions ample justice. It's amazing to experience what losing weight does for a person. It melts my heart to know that thinness is only one step away from obesity if you go down the right path.

We both competed in the race, which is a case study that most diet companies only dream of. It wasn't the first time this has happened, and in fact, there have been plenty of my diet clients who participated in athletic events right alongside their diet counselor. The success of this diet is what marketing firms wish they could brag about.

After finishing the race with a very respectable time, Andy came over to chat with me. Andrew told me that he had just returned from out of town to visit his family. The reason for the trip was to attend his aunt's funeral. He had obviously walked into a situation with a somber atmosphere, but regardless of the circumstances, the events that transpired were unexpected. His family is extremely overweight, and several of his uncles have died of heart disease. I explained to him that it's paramount to his longevity to maintain a normal body weight in order to avoid the family's maladies. The moment he entered their house, Andy felt like something was wrong. His family acted as if he had betrayed them by losing weight, because now he wasn't like the rest of the clan. There were actually members of the family who refused to hug him! One relative took his wife aside and asked her if Andy was sick. He went there expecting praise for his weight loss accomplishment, and instead he was ostracized. They gave him the cold shoulder instead of a pat on the back, and his traditional family bonding didn't occur. The next train of thought usually incites anger, because you're expecting to be complemented and that doesn't happen.

The underlying factors that contribute to this situation are not always obvious to the dieter. If you achieve success at something that others have not accomplished, the natural reaction of the underdog is jealousy. The normal weight relative now represents something they wish they could attain but haven't done so yet. Your overweight relatives now feel ashamed in your presence. When they shun you for losing weight, it's just a defense mechanism. Their actions provide them with an excuse for still being overweight. They accuse the innocent so that they don't appear guilty. When you're the pioneer of weight loss in the family, there are bound to be repercussions. You're a reminder of what they should be doing. It's as if you are their diet conscience. You used to be part of the gang, and now you are set apart because you're normal weight.

The issue here is how you overcome the peer pressure of your overweight family members. It's obvious that social gatherings usually serve food, and that's when your diet becomes more of an issue. You have to understand that just because you're in the mode of dieting doesn't mean your family wants to hear about it. If they are not psychologically ready to diet, your mere presence may upset them because they don't want to overeat in front of a victorious dieter. How you react to their remarks is important at this juncture, because it determines whether you've let them defeat you.

The best path to follow in this case is the one of least resistance. If you come off as being superior because you have done what the rest of the family doesn't have the intestinal fortitude to achieve, then you're setting yourself up for resistance and a possible ensuing argument. It's also not advisable to pass judgment upon them because this only causes feelings of resentment and shame. If you earnestly want to help your family lose weight, then use the Dale Carnegie method in this situation. It's easier to help a friend than a foe.

The key to remember now in your dieting journey is that a family is forever! It's important to maintain your composure and consider the source in this particular social situation. It's unfortunate that family members often take the liberty of saying things they shouldn't because they are, after all, your family. They hope that eventually they will be forgiven for their insensitive remarks. The optimum way to deal with the situation is to understand that people are just human and thus imperfect. If your family is jealous of you because of your weight loss, it's best not to make an issue of it and let them cool down.

If they try to encourage you to overeat, then it's time to take action. You obviously can't avoid family functions just because they are serving high-calorie food. Therefore, you should develop a plan of action before the event so that you're with your overweight family members. The way this is accomplished is by being honest with your family. Let them know that you're dieting and it's not nice to tempt you with forbidden food. It's best to call ahead and ask what's being served at the event. Then tell them that you're bringing along a great new recipe for them to enjoy. This accomplishes two things. The first of them is that now you have something to eat just in case the rest of the menu is diet unfriendly. Secondly, it allows your family to share some gourmet diet food with you, which will perhaps get them motivated enough to want to start dieting. If the topic of dieting is brought up during your conversations with the family, then use the opportunity to your advantage. If the family is inquiring about your diet, then let them know that you're in their court, and when they're ready to lose weight, you'll be their diet buddy. If your family is not cooperating with you and continues to try to sabotage your diet, then show them kindness and give them some time to adapt to the new you.

22. THE FINAL SIN

If you have ever given up any particular bad habit in life, then you'll understand exactly what this chapter's title means. There are millions of Americans who have, for instance, given up smoking cigarettes only to find solace in putting food into their mouth instead. As a result, they end up gaining weight and trading out one habit for another. When a person has decided to mend his or her ways and give up a certain activity or addiction in their life, the most common outcome is weight gain. I've put together a general list of obsessions that people quit with all good intentions and then turn to food as their companion and comforter. They are listed below:

1. Cigarettes	5. Gambling	9. Criminal Lifestyle
2. Alcohol	6. Adultery	10. Prescription Drug addiction
3. Caffeine	7. Immoral Activity	11. Gluttony - overeating
4. Drugs	8. Illicit Behavior	

The first thing that happens when you try to conquer a bad habit is the feeling of disorientation. The mere fact that you participated in this activity on a daily basis immediately alters your lifestyle. Your day-to-day actions change, and you feel like a fish out of water. Let's take the smoker as an example: the person wakes up in the morning and automatically reaches for a cup of coffee and a cigarette, then they must stop and think to themselves, "Hey, I gave up my morning cup of java and a smoke, so now what can I have?" At this point, the mind starts to go into the self-pity mode. "If I can't have my way, then I'll stop on the way to work at the donut shop and get a decaf latte and a chocolate crème-filled donut. That will make me feel better." Then the brain tries to use justification for the action. "I deserve to eat what I want because I have given up smoking, and everyone gains weight when they do so. It is expected of me." Then your thought patterns form a line of defense. "No one should have to diet and quit smoking at the same time. That is just too difficult. So why worry about the diet now? I'll take care of that later on." At this point, you have already made up your mind that it's acceptable to gain weight. The problem with this line of reasoning is that it always provides you with an excuse to overeat. This can have a domino effect because one binge leads to another, and you don't take responsibility for portion size or calorie intake. If you have no limits on the calories you ingest, your weight will rise rapidly.

There are two main reasons this type of uncontrolled eating must be avoided. The first of them occurs when you finally decide that you've gained too much weight and go on a diet; you usually discover that the damage is worse than you expected. When people are off diets, they tend to avoid the scale altogether. This results in a shock to the system as they step on the scale for their first weigh in. Then reality sets in and they realize they must lose more weight than they predicted. This means that they will have to be on a diet for a longer period of time because they let their weight creep up on them.

The second reason uncontrolled eating is adverse to successful weight loss is that you tend to develop high-calorie eating habits. I always tell my clients that you will crave what you eat. If you have been snacking on ice cream and potato chips on a regular basis, it is illogical to expect you'll get out a bag of baby carrots and munch on them instead. Once your taste buds become accustomed to high-calorie, fatty foods it will take time to acclimate them to lower-calorie food choices. Your taste buds take time to adjust to your new eating habits, and it's important to understand that you need to give yourself time to proceed and succeed.

When you are giving up a particular habit or type of lifestyle, it will not benefit you to take up overeating instead. I'll use the example of religion to make myself perfectly clear. There are many Americans that have converted to Christianity, and when they do so, they try to live a more biblical lifestyle. In an effort to clean up their lives, they give up such things as drugs, alcohol, and pornography. At this juncture in their life, they then find themselves replacing their old habits with a new habit. This new habit tends to be overeating.

The justification of this behavior is simple. The person feels that they have given up what they consider immoral, so why can't they at least eat what they want to. I'll give you a perfect example of the final sin. This client has been coming to my diet on and off for over five years. Her name is Tracy, and in her own words she doesn't drink, smoke, or party. Instead Tracy eats. As she put it, her drug of choice is food. The plain and simple fact is that people can become addicted to just about anything.

If you do something to excess and can't seem to stop once you start, then you're basically addicted. When it comes to food, it becomes difficult to discern the difference between addiction and obsession. I once had a diet client who worked as a substance abuse counselor and stated that my job was more difficult than hers. When I asked Rita why she would say such a thing, her reply was enlightening. She said that when a client came to her, they would stay at the clinic and couldn't have access to the particular drug that they were addicted to. In my case, a diet client comes to me, and I can't tell them to stop eating. They have to continue consuming food every day for the rest of their life. The person must learn to overcome a daily temptation. There are plenty of programs that try to solve this problem by designing prefabbed meals so that you don't make any choices for yourself. They sell you breakfast, lunch, and dinner and send you home with a regimented diet. There is a major flaw with this type of program. I always tell my dieters that these diets are fine for a monkey in a cage, but how does he know what to eat when you let him back out into the forest? There will be a point in time when you'll have to make up your own mind about what to eat for your three daily meals. If a program doesn't teach you how to make these decisions, the weight loss will only be temporary. If you know what foods to choose from, the knowledge stays with you for the rest of your life. You can train and condition yourself to have the self-control that you need to lose weight. This is an individual matter because each and every person has a specific reason why they overeat. The way to solve the problem is to determine the underlying factors that led to the problem.

Let's delve deeper into the life of Tracy in order to understand the true meaning of the Final Sin. As I stated earlier, she has been a client of mine for over five years. I have private diet meetings on a weekly basis so that I can develop a complete profile of each dieter in order to solve their individual weight problem. Tracy has been overweight for the majority of her life. She is 47 years old, married, and the mother of one teenage son. Tracy has tried many diets but was only willing to adhere to a program for a week and then resumed her pattern of overeating. As a result of her diet practices, she would lose 5 pounds one week and then gain 5 or 6 pounds the next week. This resulted in frustration and led her to binge more frequently.

As a result of being over 300 pounds, she had reoccurring health problems. When you have excess fat cells in your body, they provide a place for toxins to hide. The problem with obesity isn't just an issue of vanity. When you are overweight, there are always underlying health problems that occur. Tracy was constantly plagued with colds, infections, female problems, cysts, skin rashes, and heart problems that occurred. Her years of poor food choices were taking their toll on her body. Eventually Tracy developed cancer, and this became her wake up call. When you eat high-caloric food, your body becomes a storage place for hydrogenated oil, pesticides, artificial colors, and artificial flavors. The human body can only withstand so much punishment before it reacts to your bad eating habits. She decided that her life was more important than the "sinful" eating habits she had developed. The goal here is not to cop an attitude about immediate weight loss. Tracy came back with the best intentions, yet she needed to give herself some time to change her behavior. I always ask my clients, "How long did it take you to gain this weight? If it took you 30 years to develop this habit, then how can you expect to mend your ways in 2 weeks?" The only reason people desire to lose weight fast is that they want to go back to what they were eating before they started a diet. This is not the right frame of mind for dieting. The reason dieters cultivate these thoughts is because they haven't been on a real diet program. The previous diets they tried have deprived them of certain foods and even told them when and exactly what to eat, thus leaving the dieter with bad diet memories. It's time to wipe the slate clean and forget about all the other diets you were on. This program is designed to teach you how to make small dietary substitutions that lead to permanent weight loss.

When diets tell you that you must eat everything exactly according to their menu program or you will not lose weight, this is a blatant lie, or shall I say distortion of the truth. There is no magical formula that they have invented. What these books generally do is count the calories for you by providing complicated menu programs that generally add up to 1,200–1,400 calories.

Now back to Tracy. Since she was off and on the program for years, Tracy knew that the first step toward weight loss is responsibility. What I mean by this is that you should be aware of what you are eating in order to make logical changes that result in weight loss. Tracy sat down with me at her return visit to the program, and I asked her to write down what she had eaten for breakfast and lunch that day. Then I proceeded to count her calories. Tracy was aghast at the total. It was only noon, and she had already consumed 1,400 calories. When you ask a client to write down what they eat and add up their calories, it is a sobering experience. Tracy immediately saw in writing the foods that directly participated in her weight gain.

The first step toward successful weight loss is admitting how many calories you consume each day. Now you can design an individual plan of action in order to reduce your calories without deprivation. This allows you the liberty of making alterations in your diet that are livable. In some cases the changes are simple and will never alter the amount of volume you consume each day. In Tracy's case the first goal was to use less butter on her morning toast, put skim milk on her bowl of cereal, change from oil to low-calorie salad dressing on her afternoon salad, and prepare her own gourmet coffee beverage instead of stopping at a coffee house for a cup of high-calorie java. Let's take a look at how these simple substitutions add up mathematically.

TRACY'S DIET MAKEOVER

Before Diet Menu	After Diet Menu
Breakfast:	**Breakfast:**
Cereal 1 bowl	Cereal 1 bowl
Whole Milk 1 C.	Skim milk 1 C.
Coffee, cafe version	Coffee, home version
Toast 2 slices	Toast 2 slices
Butter 2 Tbsp.	Low-cal Butter 2 tsp.
	Jelly 2 tsp
Lunch: Salad	**Lunch: Salad**
Lettuce 2 C.	Lettuce 2 C.
Tomato 1 C.	Tomato 1 C.
Cucumber 1 C.	Cucumber 1 C.
Chicken 6 oz.	Carrots ½ C.
Cheese 4 oz.	Low-calorie cheese ½ oz.
Olive oil & Vinegar 4 Tbsp.	Low-calorie dressing 4 Tbsp.

Let's take a look at what these four small dietary changes yield in terms of weight loss.

Before	After	Calories saved
Coffee	**Coffee**	
Mocha Frappuccino 640 cal.	Diet version 40 cal.	600
Milk	Milk	
Whole Milk 1 C. 150 cal.	Skim Milk 90 cal.	60
Salad dressing	Salad dressing	
Olive oil and vinegar 480 cal.	Low-calorie dressing 40 cal.	440
Toast condiment	Toast condiment	
Butter, 2 Tbsp. 200 cal.	Low-calorie butter, 1 Tbsp. 50	150
	Total calories saved:	**1,250**

The above example gives you an illustration of the importance of knowing your caloric intake. If you perpetuate the caloric savings for the year, it yields 1,250 calories x 365 days, equaling 456,250 calories. The art of weight loss is accomplished by paying attention to detail! Tracy only needs to make 4 substitutions in order to lose 100 pounds!

The problem that ensues with using food as the final sin is that eating becomes uncontrolled. I'll use the example of shopping because it's something everyone can relate to. Let's say you decide to make some additions to your wardrobe. You can either set a budget limit and stick to it, or you can wave your credit card and buy anything you desire, without worrying about the debt until the credit card bill arrives in your mailbox. This can lead to financial hardships and in the extreme case even bankruptcy. This is exactly what happens with uncontrolled eating. It's just like a spending spree, except now you're on an eating spree. When you consume more calories than you burn, there will be a price to pay, similar to the credit card bills that never seem to get paid off. The calories just keep building up, and when you weigh in, your "health" statement glares at you in the form of weight gain!

You need to make up your mind when you wake up in the morning that you're going to set a budget limit on the number of calories you are going to consume. This puts you in the diet frame of mind. If you keep putting it off, it only becomes more difficult to lose weight because you've established poor eating habits that become a way of life. The justification is not valid; it's just an excuse so that you can continue your behavior without feeling guilty.

The problem with repetitive behavior is the mere fact that it's adopted as a way of life. What I mean by this is that overeating is done automatically and without forethought. The great news is that you can reverse this action and turn your bad habit into a good habit. The best way to do this is to decide in advance that you are willing to take incremental steps toward improving your eating habits.

There are two options at this juncture in your diet. The first one is not really a viable option, but it's the choice that most dieters choose. The typical dieter decides to go on a rapid weight loss program in order to reverse the damages incurred during the final sin. This is not a wise choice because it leads to frustration and sets you up for diet sabotage. When you try to give up all the wrong foods in one day, your whole way of life is disrupted. It's a drastic change that doesn't give your body or your taste buds time to adapt. It's not logical to proceed in this manner if you want to lose weight permanently. The second option is to alter your eating habits gradually so that it doesn't affect the taste or the volume of your food. This is accomplished by writing down what you eat and drink and then adding up the total net calories you consume on a daily basis. Now comes the enlightening part of the program. It's time to become your very own Diet Detective.

23. THE HOLIDAYS

As far back as I can remember, holidays weren't really about a particular day; they were about the specific food you ate on that day. This chapter is designed to provide hints and recipe suggestions for each major holiday. After reading over 100 diet books, one thing that always amazed me was that these diets don't provide a specific plan of action for each occasion. They write the book as if you're going to follow their program every day, no matter what the celebration. It's important to recognize the particular foods that tend to cause weight gain during each holiday. If you learn to make simple substitutions, you'll be able to lose or maintain your weight even during the holidays. Since we tend to be creatures of habit, why not make it a positive habit that can be used every holiday and every year?

NEW YEAR'S DAY

It's the morning after the resolution. You wake up with the notion that today will be your final binge before you start your diet. It's a bittersweet time because you know deep down inside that you made a decision that you aren't really sure you can follow through with. It's one thing to talk about dieting, and you've done plenty of that, but it's another thing to actually act upon your intention.

The thought of what the future will bring fades away when the reality of the holiday takes precedence over last night's promise. Your mind switches from pre-diet jitters to thoughts of your final day of binging. You now realize it's your last day to use the holidays as an excuse to overeat. You start to think, *it's New Year's Day, and tomorrow I'm starting my diet, so why not live it up now and eat anything I want!* You decide to finish those leftover Christmas cookies, cakes, and pies, because tomorrow you're wiping the slate clean and starting a diet.

The best way to describe this holiday is to take you back to my grandmother's house where the first feast of the year was prepared in style. As I opened the door, the scent of ham and pies swirled about the kitchen where Gram was busy making sure that all the pies were baked to perfection. The table was covered with an assortment of holiday desserts. The children would mill about the house, grabbing cookies as they passed the kitchen table. The adults sat at the table and sipped coffee and wine as they nibbled on assorted Italian cookies and desserts. It was the holiday where you could eat whatever you wanted, and no one would object or comment on your excessive caloric indulgence. The meal consisted of several main courses, which included ham, potatoes, homemade manicotti, meatballs, and pasta sauce that contained several types of meat. You were expected to save some room for Grandma's homemade pies. There were at least five different pies, and you were supposed to taste each one because you didn't want to insult the chef. If you tried to leave the table without dessert, the family treated you like a traitor.

The main problem with the New Year's Day binge is that you're eating without a dietary conscience. When you allow yourself the liberty to consume unlimited amounts of high-calorie food just because you're going on a diet the next day, you need to be aware of the repercussions that can occur as a result. The most obvious consequence is weight gain. If you try to convince yourself that you don't need to weigh in, then you're only prolonging the inevitable, which is to face what you weigh. When my clients step on the scale to begin their diet, I tell them, "This is a great day because you're facing reality, which means that you're ready to act upon your desire."

If you step on the scale one week after your New Year's binge only to find out you've maintained your weight, don't get discouraged! This is the perfect time for you to read (or reread) the Last Supper section, which explains how a final binge prior to dieting affects your first week's weigh in.

VALENTINE'S DAY

Here I sit on Valentine's Day, and my first love comes to mind. I don't mean a person either; I mean food. How many men are running out to the nearest store now, trying to fetch a "mushy" love card and a quick box of chocolates in a heart-shaped box? Even worse, how many of these men will be giving these useless calories to their overweight loved ones? That certainly doesn't express much love or gratitude. "Oh here, honey, I'm home with the forbidden fruit to help you break your diet. But after all, I bought it for you, so that makes it all right, doesn't it? One little chocolate won't hurt, will it?" The answer depends on whether it's a "danger" food for you.

It also depends on how much self-control you've had with it in the past. When my husband first met me, one thing that stuck out in his mind was when I said, "No one can make me eat anything I don't want to!" The point is to convince your brain you don't want to eat it. This will change your relationship with food. If you can feel like you're cheating and still lose weight, you won't be tempted to just give up on a whim.

Let's take a closer look at this "stuff" in the heart-shaped box. First and foremost, it has too many concentrated calories and not enough volume. It's a tease, but you can't afford to blow 300 calories on two little pieces of chocolate that weigh only a couple of ounces. Now what about the rest of the box? Who will eat the other 2,000 calories?

Secondly, a typical chocolate product contains chemicals and pesticides. Some of the worst ones can go into chocolate, because those companies save money if they believe that the buyers aren't concerned with the quality of the ingredients. There are also artificial colors, artificial flavors known to cause health problems and hydrogenated oil, which could lead to high cholesterol, arteriosclerosis, and heart disease. Therefore, that heart candy certainly won't be good for your heart.

"But Donna, what if I still want a piece of candy?" There is "bad" candy that's good for you. They taste sinful and satisfy you, but you don't wake up with yesterday's pangs of guilt. Every natural food store in this country carries a candy alternative. Even chocolate connoisseurs, who've traveled around the world just to taste chocolate, state that a natural candy bar tastes better than the ritzy-ditzy mall chocolate.

The decision still has to be made whether you want to waste 1/3 to 1/2 of your daily calories on two bites. I always ask myself, "Is it worth the calories?"

This holiday is a challenge because it doesn't just stop at the chocolates; it's by far the biggest date holiday of the year. Who would refuse a romantic evening at a fancy restaurant versus cooking? If you do decide to eat out, then plan for it in advance. If you eat 250 fewer calories for 4 days prior to the holiday, then you can enjoy 1,000 extra calories on Valentine's Day and still have the same average caloric intake. Eat slowly and enjoy your food and the company. Remember that you're there to celebrate the love that you share, not the calories. There are much better ways to celebrate love than with food, but this is a diet book, not a romance novel.

ST. PATRICK'S DAY

This is the day when everyone becomes just a little bit Irish. The traditional meal is comprised of corned beef, cabbage, and potatoes. There is only one slight problem with the meal. The protein source is extremely high in calories. Corned beef has 320 calories and 26 grams of fat for a 3-ounce portion. When you put this on a diet scale, you'll see that it's much smaller than a typical portion. The potatoes have only 100 calories per cup, and the cabbage has a measly 10 calories per cup. The plan of action is then to fill up on lower-calorie veggies and consume a small portion of the higher-calorie meat.

ST. PATRICK'S DAY DINNER

	Calories
3 ounces corned beef	320
1 C. boiled potatoes	100
3 C. boiled cabbage	30
1 slice bread	70
1 pat butter	30
Total of 550 calories	

As you can see, the total volume of this meal is over 4 ½ cups, so you should be filled up. If you still feel the urge to drink green beer, then you must decide in advance how many calories you're willing to give up in order to do so. The green beer is just a regular beer with green dye added to it, so it still has 150 calories per 12-ounce serving. You would be better off taking a light beer and putting in your own green food coloring. This will have 100 calories per 12-ounce serving. Therefore, if you have 4 light beers, you will save 200 calories. If you know that your traditional celebration involves eating out and beer drinking, then plan for it in advance. Have a low-calorie breakfast and lunch in order to save your calories for your evening out. If you do this, you won't need the "luck of the Irish" when you weigh in the next morning.

LENT

This is a time of the year to give up something we feel is important to us. It's also a time for many Americans to give up meat every Friday and eat fish or seafood instead. The problem with this dietary substitution is the method of preparation. You drive by a fish fry and there are lines going out the door. The place is swamped with people who are supposedly giving up something, and it's certainly not calories! Let me give you a perfect example of why you should not eat your seafood in the form of a fish fry. My largest diet client owned a fish fry. She ate the food there on a regular basis, and she was bigger around than she was tall. I needed two tape measures to measure her. To further illustrate my point, take a peek at the calories and fat of 5 national restaurants for a typical fish sandwich:

Restaurant	Item	Fat	Calories
Long John Silvers	Fish Meal	29	730
Burger King	Fish Sandwich	43	720
Nathans	Fillet of Fish	74	1455
Shoney's	Fish n Chips	34	639
Red Lobster	Neptunes Feast	62	1210

My heart trembles at the thought of all that fat. The problem lies in the way they cook the fish. Seafood itself is relatively low in calories. It ranges from 350 to about 800 calories per pound. It's the cooking oil that's the caloric culprit. The food is immersed and deep fried, which means the oil becomes hydrogenated. This leads to heart disease and weight gain. So, the next time you see a fish fry, drive by and do yourself a favor by eating a veggie burger instead. If you feel a need to consume seafood, then save yourself hundreds of calories and prepare it at home in the oven without the added fat and calories. You will be able to eat more volume and fewer calories, which in turn yields weight loss.

EASTER

Did you ever notice that just the mention of a holiday brings about a food thought? You mention Easter, and people think of ham and chocolate. If you have children, the day starts with your youngsters opening the Easter basket and munching on an assortment of their favorite sweets. I recommend that you purchase candy that you don't like and put it in your children's Easter baskets. This prevents the "Easter raid" as I call it. How many clients have gained weight the week after Easter because they've seized their children's Easter candy? This way you won't be tempted to eat what you don't like. If your children prefer the same sweets that you do, then put healthier versions of candy in their basket. I find an organic candy bar tastes so much better than the run-of-the-mill chocolate; therefore you'll be satisfied with eating less of it. Try putting some nuts, seeds, and dried fruit into their basket. This will teach them better eating habits and help control everyone's weight.

Following the candy is the Easter dinner. This usually involves ham, potatoes, a vegetable, and assorted pies and desserts. The plan of action is to consume less of the high-calorie food and more of the low-calorie food. If the dinner involves ham, you should keep in mind that it has 100 calories per ounce. The potatoes have only 100 calories per cup. If they're mashed potatoes, remember that the milk and butter used in the recipe add more calories than the potato itself. The desserts are the part of the meal where discretion is important. The highest calorie part of the pie is the crust, which is comprised of lard and flour. Keep in mind that a typical piece of pie has 500 calories. The lower-calorie pies are pumpkin and lemon, while the higher-calorie ones are pecan and chocolate. If you eat the pie without the crust, it has only 250–300 calories. Let's take a look at a typical Easter menu and add up the calories of the dinner.

REVISED EASTER MENU

	Calories
3 oz. lean ham	300
1 C. mashed potatoes w/butter & milk	200
2 oz. gravy prepared with water	25
1 C. vegetables	50
1 tsp. butter	30
1 slice apple pie without crust	300
Total 905 calories	

If you prepare the Easter dinner, give the leftover pies and sweets to your friends and relatives to take home or freeze the remains for future use. It's important that you keep food out of sight. I have always said, "Out of sight, out of mind." Who wants to open the refrigerator the next morning and see five different leftover pies staring them in the face? You might just find yourself eating some for breakfast.

The children's baskets should be kept in their rooms so that you're not tempted to pick up a piece of candy. As you pass by, remind yourself that the goal is to lose weight. You can consume 500 calories in candy in 5 minutes. To put this into perspective, think of it this way: you would have to run 5 miles just to burn off those 500 calories; and then you would only be back to even. Ask yourself if the calories are worth it *before* you eat the food, not afterward. Think of the real reason for celebrating Easter and be thankful for the blessings that you have in life!

MOTHER'S DAY

This is your (or your wife's) special day. A time when families come together to appreciate a mother's years of devotion and unconditional love for them. What kind of a family would make Mom cook on Mother's Day? I realize that everyone needs a break from their daily routine, and treating you to dinner is the family's way of telling you to go ahead, relax and enjoy your holiday. Once again, if you know that you will be eating out, just plan for it in advance. (See The Dieter's Guide to Dining Out.) It's a good idea to tell your family in advance that you're dieting. Ask them to purchase non-food gifts. A gift certificate to a stylish clothing store would be a suitable idea, since you will need a smaller size wardrobe.

FATHER'S DAY

This is Dad's special day. It's a time of year to show your heartfelt appreciation of his years of love and affection. If your father is overweight, don't tempt him with high-calorie foods that will result in weight gain. If your Mom is on a diet, or you are, then don't put the family in a position of having to binge because the food was just there. This holiday is often celebrated by eating at a restaurant, but you can cook a special meal for your father or husband, one that contains low-calorie options and enjoy the celebration. Don't give food as a gift to a dieter. The temptation is overwhelming, and sometimes a binge becomes an excuse to stop dieting completely. Remember that the real reason for the day is to honor your father, not food!

MEMORIAL DAY, JULY 4TH, LABOR DAY (ALSO PICNICS AND BARBECUES)

Summer is a time of outdoor barbecues, family picnics, and trips to the Local Park or beach. The mere mention of a summer holiday brings to mind hamburgers, hot dogs, and macaroni salad. Many dieters find it difficult to adhere to their program on such days. The most important thing is to make up your mind before you attend the social event that dieting is more important to you than overeating. Listed below are the holiday hints you should read before each summer party.

HOLIDAY HINTS

Remember to bring low-calorie dressing with you on your picnic.

- Regular salad dressing: 1 Tbsp . . . . 90 calories
- Low-calorie salad dressing: 1 Tbsp. . . . 20 calories

Prepare low-calorie salads ahead of time and bring them with you (see Quick Salad Ideas).

- 1 C. regular potato salad . . . . 500 calories
- 1 C. low-calorie potato salad . . . . 140 calories
- Do not eat salads made with regular mayonnaise or oil.
- 1 Tbsp. mayonnaise . . . . 100 calories
- 1 Tbsp. oil . . . . 120 calories

If you consume alcohol, then drink low-calorie beer or alcohol with diet soda.

- Example: 5 light beers = 500 calories
- Omit Meal 1 and snack

After dinner, take a walk. This will boost your metabolism and get you away from the table.

Don't let yourself be talked into overeating.

Walk away from any food that you can't stop eating once you start.

Don't eat just because you see other people eating. Keep yourself busy and remember that the goal is to lose weight, not gain it. While others are eating, play some games instead, like softball, horseshoes, jarts, badminton, or frisbee.

MEMORIAL DAY, JULY 4TH, AND LABOR DAY MENU PLAN

Meal 1:	Net Calories
1 piece of fruit (your choice)	50
1 piece diet bread, toasted	40
1 tsp. low-calorie jelly	<u>15</u>
50 calorie fruit ideas:	**105**
1 small apple, 1 C. berries, 1 C. cantaloupe, 1 grapefruit, 1 C. grapes, 1 C. honeydew, 2 peaches, 1 small pear, 1 orange, 1 C. pineapple, 2 C. watermelon	

Meal 2:	
1 fat-free or vegetarian frankfurter	45
1 low-calorie hot dog roll	100
1 Tbsp. mustard	6
1 tsp catsup	10
1 dill pickle	5
1 serving low-calorie macaroni salad	<u>161</u>
(see Quick Salad Ideas)	**327**
Deluxe Tossed Salad	5
1 c. lettuce	20
1 tomato, chopped	15
1 cucumber, chopped	5
¼ C. mushrooms, sliced	5
¼ C. green peppers, chopped	10
¼ C. onions, chopped	<u>60</u>
3 Tbsp. low-calorie salad dressing	**120**
	Total = 447

Meal 3:	
Deluxe Cheeseburger	
¼ lb. lean ground beef (4 oz.)	280
1 low-calorie hamburger roll, or whole wheat	100
1 slice low-calorie cheese	50
1 tsp. mustard	6
1 tsp. catsup	10
2 onion slices	5
2 tomato slices	5
½ C. lettuce	2
1 pickle, sliced	5
1 serving creamy potato salad (see Quick Salad Ideas)	140
1 serving macaroni salad (see Quick Salad Ideas)	<u>160</u>
(Spread mustard and catsup on hamburger roll, add cheeseburger, top with onion, tomato, pickles, and lettuce.)	**763**

Meal 4: Snack	
1 oz. low-calorie potato crisps	90
1 oz. nonfat tortilla chips	110
2 oz. salsa	5
1 slice watermelon	<u>50</u>
	255

| **Total calories for the day** | **1570** |

HALLOWEEN

This is a holiday that can sabotage any diet. The main reason is that the candy is simply in the house and accessible to the dieter before, during, and after the holiday. How many times have I heard the horror story (no, this is not an urban legend; it's the truth) of a client who buys the candy in advance and ends up eating it all before Halloween even arrives! The simple way to avoid this pitfall is to wait until Halloween to buy the candy. I recommend you purchase a type of candy to pass out that you will not eat yourself. Why would you be buying candy you like? In order to please some children knocking at your door for free treats? I sense an ulterior motive!

If you'll be taking your children out to trick-or-treat and any of them are overweight, then it's your responsibility to provide lower-calorie options so the holiday doesn't bring on more weight. If you traditionally go out to collect candy for two hours, then limit the kids to ten houses and provide some natural sweets at home in order to continue the celebration. Make a homemade batch of fat-free brownies to warm up to when you get home. It's important to instill good eating habits when the kids are young. You know how difficult it can be to change a 20-year habit! The less candy they come home with, the fewer calories they will consume.

Another option is to host a costume party for the children and provide low-calorie treats such as old-fashioned candied apples or low-fat cupcakes. Plan activities that don't involve food. Rent an old-fashioned monster movie and relax to a fresh bowl of popcorn. This is a perfect time to teach your children that candy is not a fifth food group. The calories are so concentrated that most candy bars have 150 calories per ounce! *The best way to lead is by example.* So, show your loved ones that there is more to Halloween than just sweets.

THANKSGIVING

This is the day that dieting is often the farthest thing from your mind. After all, this is the start of the holidays, and you'll be going on a weight loss program after New Year's, so party on! The problem with this concept is simple. It's not as easy to lose weight as it is to gain weight. Wouldn't it be nice if you could eat more selectively and maintain your weight? Listed below are tips that teach you how to eat more volume and fewer calories on turkey day.

The right-hand side of the list is provided for the dieter who is preparing the Thanksgiving feast. It's a list of simple substitutions that will save you over a thousand calories. The changes I've suggested will not alter the taste or volume of your dinner!

Traditional Preparation		Reduced-calorie Preparation
If your family serves the traditional cheese, crackers, chips, veggies, and dip, the best plan of action is to eat more vegetables and a couple of crackers and cheese. Stay away from the dip, which can be as high as 100 calories per ounce. Olives are a nice substitute because they are only 5-10 calories each. Omit regular cheese and choose a gourmet cheese that is stronger in taste and more robust in flavor. You tend to eat less of things that have texture and flavor.	Appetizers	Omit regular sour cream or cream cheese from your dip and use low-fat sour cream or low-fat cream cheese.

Omit high-fat crackers and use a gourmet type cracker or flavored cracker that adds flare to your appetizer tray.

Omit high-fat chips and have a unique chip like sweet potato chips or blue corn chips and a mango peach salsa.

Omit run-of-the-mill canned black olives. Buy an imported stuffed olive. They are so tasty you will be satisfied after the first bite. I have tasted olives from Greece stuffed with feta cheese that provide more flavor than a whole jar of ordinary green olives. |
	Main Entree	
	Turkey	Choose the breast or white meat without skin. This is only 60 calories per ounce.
You should be aware that dressing is prepared with a stick of butter so it can be high in fat as well as calories. Go light on this and save some calories.	Stuffing	Omit the butter and substitute a tad more broth. Add vegetables such as mushrooms and onions for a gourmet touch.
Most chefs prepare them with milk and butter, but they are still much lower in calories than a dessert.	Mashed Potatoes	Omit the butter and use light butter.

Omit the whole milk and use skim milk. |
| If the gravy is prepared with the juice from the turkey, then it can be more calories than it looks. | Gravy | Omit the meat drippings and use water instead. |

The yam itself is only 70 net calories per C. The culprit here is the condiments. If they top it with butter, that adds 120 cal. per tablespoon. If it is candied, the sweetener is approximately 50 calories per tablespoon.	Sweet Potatoes or Yams	Cook without butter and top with low-calorie butter and a low-calorie sweetener
Veggies are a dieter's best friend. The average calories per C. are only 50 net calories. Once again, the condiment contributes the majority of the calories. If you add oil, margarine, or butter, keep in mind one small teaspoon is 33 calories.	Cooked Vegetables	Omit the butter, margarine, and oil and instead bake or broil them with special seasonings for a holiday treat.
Pumpkin pie is the lowest calorie pie, and the filling also contains fiber. The highest calorie part of any pie is the crust, so eat only half the crust and save calories. Keep in mind a small piece of pie is still around 500 calories.	Dessert	Prepare a pie using a low-calorie crust. If the pie has a pudding filling, use water or skim milk to prepare the filling instead of whole milk. Prepare a fat-free brownie and top with low-fat ice cream and fat-free fudge topping. Surprise the family with a new gourmet diet dessert
This is not the day to waste calories on liquids unless they are worth it. Remember that regular soda contains 150 calories per 12 ounce serving. If you decide to drink alcohol, then be aware of the fact that cordials and liqueurs are the higher calorie alcoholic beverages. Stay away from prepared drink mixes. There can be up to 500 calories in just the mixer. Prepare your own. They always taste better, and at least you know what goes into it.	Beverages	Omit regular soda and have diet soda or seltzer instead. Use low-calorie mixers for alcoholic beverages. Omit regular beer and drink light beer instead. Add some zero-calorie flavored seltzer to your wine to cut the calories and make it last longer.

THE HOLIDAY SEASON

There are about 40 days between Thanksgiving and the beginning of a New Year's resolution. If you eat only 500 more calories each day, this can put on 5 ¾ pounds before you even know it. I know that 500 calories sounds like a lot, but it really means only 2 extra Christmas cookies or a sliver of pie and a cocktail at the company Christmas party.

Many dieters don't weigh themselves during this time because they would rather not know the facts and figures. *You need to face the scale in order to change the scale.* In this case, ignorance is not bliss. In fact, it might just turn into depression if you don't confront the issue and deal with it in a suitable manner.

Weight loss is within your reach as long as the program is something you can live with daily. So, don't get upset and think that I'm asking you to ruin your favorite binge time of year. The best gifts you can give your family are longevity and good health, which go hand in hand with weight loss.

The main reason people decide not to diet during holidays is that it's not the appropriate or popular thing to do. After all, everyone else is having a jolly old time eating anything they want, so why can't I? The first thing I learned to do, in order to be a successful dieter, is to never let other people determine what I eat. The social pressure is evident at every joyous occasion and therefore must be dealt with on a daily basis. Remember that the people who prod you to eat won't have to squeeze into their jeans tomorrow morning, nor do they have to feel guilty when you weigh in!

It's important that *you* decide what you eat, when you eat, and how much you eat. Discipline goes a long way, and with practice, it's something that becomes a good habit. You can be proud of yourself after the party, and you can also be an example for other dieters to follow in your weight-loss footsteps. You don't have to sit at a Christmas party and munch on celery sticks and drink seltzer water, but the behavior that led to last year's holiday weight gain must be changed.

Now let's discuss little changes that you can employ during the holidays. The first thing to be changed is your mind. I always tell my clients, "If you can perceive it, you can achieve it." You need to make up your mind that this season will not result in weight gain. Maintaining your current weight is better than gaining weight.

I recommend that you write down what you eat, even if you don't count your calories. This gives you a record of the events, as well as holding you responsible for what you consume. If you can't do such a thing at this time of year, then meet me halfway and at least choose a strategy you can live with.

THE CHRISTMAS PARTY

The purpose of any party is to socialize and enjoy the evening, not to gain weight. Here are some tips:

- One option is to eat at least 200 fewer calories for two days prior to the event, so you bank up 400 calories. Then you can afford to eat 400 extra calories the day of the party.

- If you drink alcohol at the party, be sure to have a no-calorie or low-calorie mixer. Diet soda or spritzers are the perfect choice. If you're having wine, the 20 calories per ounce can easily last longer with diet spritzer added to them. If you're consuming beer, make sure it's light in calories. Some sneaky companies call their beer light when it has 136 calories (compared to a regular beer with 150 calories). So, choose a light beer that's got between 95 and 110 calories per bottle.

- At the buffet table, try to avoid sauces, dips, and condiments that are high in calories and fat. For example, there's no harm in 10 baby carrots, which equal about 10 calories, but that thick ranch dressing will add about 150 calories to the innocent vegetables. Start by munching on raw fruit and vegetables, because they take a long time to eat. After the low-calorie appetizers have diminished your hunger, you can try a higher-calorie food, but eat only half as much as you normally would.

- You should make up your mind that you'll stop eating when you reach your caloric limit. Watch out for your danger foods, which are substances that you can't stop eating, no matter how many times you've told yourself that you've had enough! If you find your favorite dessert is sitting there looking pretty and calling your name, then maybe it's better not to take the first bite at all. Is it really worth the 5 minutes of pleasure only to find out the next day that you have gained weight? Don't let a temptation get in the way of your achievement. There is no better feeling than overcoming your dietary weakness and waking up in the morning with pride and dignity instead of hating yourself for your minor setbacks.

- Another practice helping me stay thin is that I don't feel a responsibility to eat all the food on my plate. If you feel guilty about throwing food in the garbage, then why are you throwing it down your throat? As I told one of my clients at their diet meeting, "You already paid for the food, therefore the money is spent, so what are you really saving?" Absolutely nothing, and in turn you're now making your body the garbage can. If you still feel that you can't bring yourself to "waste" the food, then put it outside and let some poor squirrel put on his winter fat, or put it in a bird feeder and enjoy the show.

A little self-control, or lack thereof, can go a long way. Year after year, I hear my dieters say that they only have a small piece of pie or a couple holiday cookies or a few chocolates. Okay, but it doesn't take much high-calorie food to pack on the pounds. If you only ate a little, then why are you finding that you weigh increasingly more year after year? The answer is in the all-important calorie. If you have a tiny plate with some cookies, pie, or chocolate, it won't look like you're eating much. However, volume isn't the deciding factor; calories are. You can gain a lot of weight from eating small portions, if those portions are very high in calories. On the other hand, if you eat the right foods, your serving size can be much bigger! As for me, I'd rather have a fulfilling plate of fruit and raw veggies with 50–100 calories instead of a 100-calorie cookie that would be gone in just one bite.

HOLIDAY EGGNOG

Now that we're on the topic of the holiday eating spree, there's one more item that needs to be discussed, that once-in-a-year seasonal item called eggnog. Much to my surprise, the grocery and convenience store version of eggnog has 450 calories per 8-ounce serving and 26 grams of fat. If you indulge in only a small cup per day between Thanksgiving and New Year's Day, you will add 18,000 extra calories to your diet and up to 5 pounds of weight to your waistline. That's without adding any extra items such as alcohol. Now take a look at the figures for a cup of eggnog with rum, vodka, or another alcohol every day. That adds to 450 calories for the eggnog and 100 calories for the alcohol, for a total of 550 calories. So, forget the eggnog or make your own low-calorie version of the classic Christmas beverage.

CHRISTMAS DAY

So this is Christmas, a day steeped in tradition and rituals for over 2,000 years. It's slightly easier than Thanksgiving for a dieter, because the primary attention is usually focused on opening your gifts. There's hardly a better gift to give yourself and your family than weight loss. When you achieve a goal in the midst of temptation and against all odds, it boosts your self-esteem. After all, if you can lose weight during the holidays, you can do it anytime of the year.

I'm fully aware that tradition plays a major role in the food you prepare and serve. One of my client's families has been eating the same menu for 57 years. If this sounds like your family, there are a few options available. One is to bring a new recipe that everyone will love. Why not start a new tradition, one that you can be proud of, because it doesn't contribute to obesity? I don't have the heart to prepare a high-calorie dessert or meal for an overweight person. Don't contribute to the problem; instead help them solve it. Even if you simply reduce the calories from one of the family's all-time favorites, you'll still be taking steps that result in weight loss. With small substitutions, you'll have the same volume and taste of your favorite foods.

Another option is to bank up your calories for that day. This is premeditated binging. You know you will eat more calories that day than you should, so use math to your advantage. Eat 500 fewer calories for 2 days prior. This saves you 1,000 calories, so you can consume 1,000 more calories on Christmas Day.

Above all, instead of concentrating on food this holiday, spend some time thinking about the true meaning of *Christ*mas.

THE BUFFET TABLE

Now it's time to study the buffet table, which usually consists of hot and cold items. First let's take an intricate look at the luncheon meat tray. The usual fare includes turkey, roast beef, ham, American cheese, and rolls, with condiments to accompany them. The choice you make at this juncture can save you hundreds of calories. The lowest calorie cold cut is the turkey breast. It has only 50 calories per ounce versus the roast beef, which has 100. You probably aren't carrying your diet scale to the party, so you'll need a way to estimate the weight of your luncheon meat. The easiest way is to compare it to the average deli slice, which has one ounce, so gauge your portions in this manner. If you add 1 slice of cheese, remember that it's got about 100 calories per ounce, so choose a slice of something you really enjoy.

Then there's the roll. In order to estimate the calories, think of it this way: a single slice of regular bread has 70 calories per slice. Next, come the typical condiments, which can add more calories to the sandwich than everything else inside it. Mayonnaise and dips have 100 calories per tablespoon, while mustard has only 10. If the thought of a mustard sandwich has your stomach churning, then why not try my technique, and walk over to the vegetable platter and munch on the carrots, broccoli, and tomatoes with your sandwich. The whole concoction tastes much more appealing and saves between 200–300 calories. *Why waste a calorie if you can barely taste a calorie?* The revised diet sandwich calories then add up to the following: dinner roll or 2 slices of bread are 140, 2 slices of turkey meat are 100, raw veggies are only 10, for a total of 250 calories.

Let's move on to the hot section of the buffet. If it's an upscale style menu, you may see ham, roast beef, turkey, and a seafood selection. The lowest calorie choice in this case is seafood. Shrimp that isn't breaded is the wise choice because it contains only 20 calories per ounce versus beef or ham, which tip the scale at 100 calories per ounce. You should be beware of the condiments that accompany seafood, such as white or butter sauce, which have about 100 calories per tablespoons Hidden calories are unfortunate because the scale doesn't forget them. Most holiday fare includes a pasta-baked casserole, which is fine as long as you don't see fat floating on top. The fat indicates that the recipe is cooked with oil or butter, which are calories that don't add volume to your diet. Eggplant Parmesan is a perfect example of a vegetable gone astray. The eggplant itself contains only 20 calories per cup, but deep fry this innocent veggie in oil, add bread crumbs, and then pile cheese on it, and it'll have about 400 calories per cup! A suitable pasta casserole is one that contains pasta, ricotta, and cheese. The damages for a cup of baked pasta are about 300 calories, and even less if you spare the cheese. Remember to eat slowly and enjoy each and every bite you get. Even the most discerning dieter will have to use self-control and wisdom when attending a social event.

Now we turn our sight to the dessert section of the table. Now think about this: each small cookie can range from 200 - 400 calories each. Will you be able to eat just one and stop? Most of my clients can't. The best plan of action is to fill your plate with the acceptable foods and walk away. You're there to have a good time and socialize. My friends and relatives say I talk more than I eat. I'm very thankful for this habit and suggest you do the same thing!

Finally, in order to curb your hunger and prevent poor food choices, fill up your hand with a low-calorie beverage. The holidays will come every year, so the time to make a positive change is now. It's much easier to gain weight than it is to lose weight. Don't put yourself in a position that yields failure or guilt. Leave room for success and happiness. Stop letting other people talk you into eating food just because they're eating it. They don't have to live inside your body, and it doesn't make any logical sense to gain weight just because you wanted to eat what your overweight friends and family are consuming. Misery loves company! *I say success loves company!* Your life will be changing as you lose weight, and those social prompts will be a thing of the past. Don't let anyone get in the way of your weight loss. Learn to say "No thank you!"

THE CHEAT WEEK

The cheat week starts on Christmas Eve and it stops the day after New Year's. The most common New Year's resolution in America is obviously to go on a diet. During cheat week, I notice an unusual amount of traffic at every fast-food joint and restaurant in our town. I know exactly what's going on: the last minute binges during the final week of eating anything the heart desires. This is justified in a dieter's mind because after the New Year they'll be depriving themselves of forbidden foods. So why not live it up now? The problem with this is that you crave what you eat. If you start the day with a donut, how do you expect to suddenly wake up in seven days to an apple and a whole grain English muffin? What if the next diet week never comes? Even the best diet intentions go astray when an opportunity comes along to binge. The ability to achieve successful and permanent weight loss lies in the fact that my diet is one that you can follow every day. Besides, if you cheat and end up gaining 3–5 pounds of fat that week, it could take you up to 1 full month to lose it. Ask yourself, "Is it worth the price you pay?"

When it comes to weight loss, this advice is worth its weight in gold: if you don't gain it, you don't have to lose it. Try eating only half of the high-calorie foods that you usually eat. Make a commitment to yourself that you can keep. I ask my clients, "Is it really worth the 5–10 minutes of so-called pleasure to blow your diet for the whole day?"

The year concludes with the New Year's Eve celebration. If yours is filled with traditional drinks and feasting, then you must plan your dieting strategy in advance. You know that there will be appetizers, food, and drinks, and you'll have to stay up until the ball drops, so that's more hours of eating than usual. Just remember that you can always offset that late-night eating by reducing 300 or more calories from other meals before the social occasion.

TODAY IS YOUR BIRTHDAY

As I write this, today is my birthday. In fact, every entry in the holiday chapter has been written on the actual holiday, to capture the truths of each event. There is no substitute for reality. Today I ponder my previous birthday experiences and how my eating habits and desires have changed. The one particular event that sticks in my mind is the obligatory birthday party, which leads to blowing out my candles, which by now would probably be considered a fire hazard, because so many of them are lit simultaneously. I say this only in jest, because I'm blessed to be able to celebrate each year with increased vitality. It's a fact that you can increase your longevity and age with grace. (This subject matter is discussed in detail in the section entitled what's My Bonus?) Now, back to the typical birthday decision: "Do I eat the cake or politely refuse to have a piece of my own birthday cake?" The snack appears innocent, but it can affect the very outcome of one's present body weight.

I'm not saying that you need to lose weight because you ate a piece of your birthday cake. What I'm stating is that your cake probably wasn't the only piece you've had all year long. You celebrate the birthdays of your family, friends, and co-workers. Then there are the anniversary parties, graduations, weddings, and baby showers, retirement celebrations, and weddings, not to mention the traditional holidays that include eating cake as part of the festivities. It all begins to add up, and before you know it, you're eating a piece of cake almost every week.

This chapter is not written in order to rain on your birthday. I'm putting my pencil to paper in order to instruct you as to how you can have a great birthday without gaining weight. The goal is to lose weight, and you shouldn't lose sight of that every time a holiday or social event comes your way.

Listed below are tips that allow you to celebrate your special day without gaining weight.

DIETER'S GUIDE TO ENJOYING A HAPPY BIRTHDAY!

You could reduce your caloric intake by 100 calories daily for five days before your birthday. This gives you some calorie leeway in case you consume extra calories at your birthday party.

If you know that you're going out to dinner or attending a birthday bash, then before your social event, eat a light breakfast and lunch, adding up to less than 300 calories.

If you're hosting your own party, take the time to prepare a gourmet diet cake. It will not only benefit your weight loss endeavors, but it will also help other guests that are dieting. If you need assistance for making a low-calorie dessert, see the chapter on Breaking the Rules. If you're hesitating to alter your traditional cake recipe, then ponder the fact that a typical piece of cake has over 600 calories!

If you plan to drink alcohol, then reduce the calories of your food to offset those from your cocktails. This aspect of dieting is also discussed in detail in Breaking the Rules!

The perfect gift to give yourself on your birthday is a good workout. It's an ingenious idea because it burns some of the day's increased calories and puts you into a dieting frame of mind. This in turn gives you a sense of accomplishment and builds your self-esteem.

You should inform your guests that you would prefer that they give you non-food gifts. *The less temptation, the less condemnation.* You don't need extra high-calorie food in your home, luring you into eating just because you feel obligated to use your present.

It's a perfect day to savor the flavor of a gourmet appetizer tray. The platter should consist of assorted fruits like grapes, strawberries, and melons. They go perfectly with an array of gourmet cheeses from around the world. It's always interesting to try several new cheeses, which will expand your food horizons. The best way to serve your specialty cheese is with a unique selection of whole grain crackers. If you take a trip to your local gourmet health food store, you'll be pleasantly surprised at the selection of high fiber crackers. There are plenty of new snack items, such as spelt crackers and multi-grain flats. Blue corn chips add color and flair to your appetizer tray, and they pair well with all types of cheese. If you're in the mood for munching, then adorn your platter with roasted red or yellow peppers, artichoke hearts, and gourmet stuffed olives. If the marinated items are packed in oil, drain it off before serving to remove all the tasteless calories.

Don't let your family and friends coerce you into eating food that you weren't planning to eat. The justification, "Oh, it's your birthday, go ahead and have another piece of cake," could lead to dietary disaster. You can always find a reason to overeat if you really want to. Don't let excuses determine your behavior. Instead, focus on what you want to weigh on your next birthday. You should apply a positive train of thought such as, *it's my birthday, and I'm going to lose weight so that I can enjoy more birthdays, because I'll be living longer!*

If you don't write down what you eat on your birthday because you're ashamed or you don't want to think about how many calories there were, then it's time to get back in the diet saddle again. The most important thing you can do is to start again the next day, writing down what you eat and counting your net calories. Don't let time lapse, because it will only become more difficult to get back in the habit of completing your food and beverage journal.

Here's another trick I pull out of my dietary arsenal, which is especially good for birthdays. If you're concerned with good health and longevity, it's time to look at food for what it really is! If something has the skull and crossbones on the label, you wouldn't eat or drink it, would you? Some foods should really have that symbol, considering the health problems they cause. Suppose someone asked you to eat food with artificial flavors and colors (which could cause cancer) and hydrogenated oils (which cause heart disease) and processed sugar (which causes diabetes). You would reply with a stern, "No, of course I wouldn't eat that!" Well then, the next time you're at a birthday party, you had better say "No" to the birthday cake, because that was the food I just described. Ask yourself if it's worth the damage! Our culture has a habit of making sweets appear so pretty and colorful. Eat with your brain first and your eyes last. Remember what the food is really made of, and it will become an appetite suppressant instead of a lure that snags you in the end.

24. DIETER'S GUIDE TO DINING OUT

When you call your favorite establishment to make reservations, ask them the specifics of the entrée you will be ordering. Chefs are proud to offer their specialty items with a minute change that renders them a diet meal.

1. If you are having a salad with your dinner, order it with low-calorie dressing on the side. If you do not, you will be wasting over 500 calories in the salad dressing, while the salad itself is only 75 calories. If the restaurant doesn't have diet dressing, then you can bring your own low-calorie one, or use theirs sparingly and add some vinegar to it.

2. If you order grilled fish or seafood, ask for it to be cooked dry. This will save you about 500 calories because the oil or butter is simply taken out of the recipe.

3. Do not order food that is cooked in cream or white sauces.

4. Do not order deep-fried appetizers or deep-fried dinners. Even eggplant becomes high in calories when it turns into Eggplant Parmesan.

5. Do not order rice in the form of pilafs. That usually means cooked in a lot of butter or oil.

6. Do order a baked potato and make sure the butter and sour cream are put on the side. The reason I'm firm on this is that most restaurants put a scoop of butter on the potato when it's hot, and you won't even know how many hidden calories have melted into your innocent potato. Remember the potato is 90 calories; the scoop of butter is 250 calories!

7. Do order a low-calorie protein source such as seafood, chicken, turkey, or a vegetarian alternative. The preferred method of low-calorie preparation is broiled dry, baked, or grilled without the skin and fat trimmed off.

8. Do order a low-calorie beverage such as sparkling water or diet soda or a low-calorie alcoholic beverage. Don't order alcohol with cream or regular soda. Instead, ask for diet soda as a mixer. Liqueur and cordials are all over 100 calories per ounce. So avoid them, or once again make sure that it's worth the calories.

9. Refrain from dessert. You probably are up to your caloric limit anyway. If you must order it, then ask for a bowl of fresh fruit, or order one dessert and share it with someone at your table.

10. Don't let your dining partner(s) influence your menu choices.

SALAD WITH BREAD OR ROLLS:

- Bring your own salad dressing or ask for low-calorie salad dressing. Make sure your salad dressing is always ordered on the side so that you are aware of how much you put on your salad.

- Have one (1) piece of bread or a small dinner roll. Remember that each pat of butter is 33 calories.

APPETIZER:

- Stay away from all deep-fried choices. They can have more calories than your main entrée. A shrimp cocktail is one of the lowest calorie choices. It's best to save your calories for the dinner.

- Many dieters have gone astray with what seems to be an innocent bowl of soup. One of the all-time favorites is French Onion Soup. What's the harm in that? It's probably only a couple of wholesome onions put into a simple broth. Let's take a closer look at this bowl of so-called safe soup. It usually contains pieces of crusty bread that were probably browned in butter and then topped with Swiss cheese. The calories can range from 300–600, which is far too many to waste on one bowl of soup. Stay away from creamed soups because they could actually be prepared with heavy cream, which has 100 calories per ounce. Once again, these types of soups can be as high as 500 calories per serving.

CARBOHYDRATE:

There are usually four types of carbohydrates to choose from, which are potatoes, rice, pasta, and pizza. Let's take a closer look at our individual options.

POTATO:

- Worst Choices: French Fries, AuGratin, Twice Baked
- Best Choices: Steamed, Broiled, Baked (sour cream and butter on the side)

RICE:

- Worst Choices: Rice Pilaf, Pork Fried Rice
- Best Choices: Steamed, Spanish Rice

PASTA:

- Worst Choices: Alfredo, White Clam Sauce, cream or butter sauces
- Best Choices: Marinara Sauce

PIZZA:

- Worst Choices: Pizza from large franchises that use oil in the sauce, in the dough, and on the pan; pizzas cooked in pans; white pizza (the sauce is usually oil!)
- Best Choices: Pizza made from flour, H_2O, yeast, and salt with crushed tomato sauce and low-fat Mozzarella
- Worst Toppings: Beef, sausage, ham
- Best Toppings: Pepperoni (only because they don't put many slices on) and all vegetables that are put on fresh and/or are canned without the addition of oil.

PROTEIN:

- The caloric density of protein may vary from 30 calories per ounce for tofu up to 100 calories per once for pork, beef, and ham.
- Worst Choices: Prime Rib, pork chops, hamburgers, hot dogs, chicken wings, ribs, roast beef, sausage, pork loin, ham, and bacon
- Best Choices: Chicken and or turkey breast, vegetarian burger, tofu, seafood, both fresh water and salt water fish

CONDIMENTS:

- Stay away from sauces that use oil, butter, cream, or cheese as their base; instead order a sauce that is derived from a vegetable like soy sauce or marinara sauce. Hidden fat calories add up quickly. Remember that oil, butter, and cream all have 120 calories per tablespoon, and that's only 3 measly teaspoons.

25. THE GRAND FINALE

A diet isn't just a program; it's a lifestyle. That's why the only diet I offer you is one that you can live with for the rest of your life. In this chapter, I'll help you recognize when you've arrived at a weight that you're happy with. Also more importantly, I'll show you how to maintain your slimmer shape—and healthier lifestyle—for as long as you live.

It's a typical question among my diet clients: "What should my goal weight be?" It was a common practice of diet companies to determine your "ideal" weight by using the standard height and weight charts. This methodology can be used as a guideline, but it has some major problems:

- It doesn't take into account your percentage of body fat.

- It was originally designed to qualify a person to receive a life insurance policy. If your weight was over their chart's maximum limit, the applicant was denied the policy.

- You can misjudge which body frame category you fall into. It's comforting to think you're a large frame, because now you can weigh more and the chart indicates you're "normal" weight.

The justification for your current body weight should not be the basic life insurance weight and height chart. Instead, I tell my clients to stand naked in a full-length mirror and turn around slowly until they face the mirror again. If there's a smile on their face, then they are at their goal weight. The whole issue of a particular number on the scale puts the dieter under unnecessary stress and pressure. They anticipate that when they reach a magical number that they're aiming for, they'll look exactly the way they want. The obsession with one number is not conducive to permanent weight loss, because the dieter is constantly putting him or herself on trial. If he doesn't achieve the ultimate weight he wants to weigh, then it's human nature for him to give up all together. When he feels that the goal is no longer attainable, the "why bother" attitude tends to take over.

The best way to achieve permanent weight loss is to allow yourself space to succeed. If you plan on losing the most possible weight in the least amount of time, then you're setting yourself up to quit the diet, because it didn't meet up to your expectations. When you take time to give yourself credit for your diet accomplishments, your frame of mind changes, and weight loss becomes a natural transition instead of a test.

THE BIG DAY

So now comes the big day when you look in the mirror and you're smiling. You actually look forward to weighing in, because you want to know how much weight you've lost. The first thought that goes through your mind is, *Ah, I've lost the weight and I can finally stop dieting!* It's fine to savor the moment, but don't put yourself into a non-dieting frame of mind so quickly. I understand why this notion pops up, but one detail that needs to be addressed is *weight maintenance.* The most sinful diet myth ever written is that you can go back to eating your normal diet and still maintain your weight loss because now your metabolism is boosted and you burn more calories than before. The exact statement may vary from publication to publication, but the gist is still the same. If you wonder why so many dieters gain all their weight back and the success rate for permanent weight loss is at an all-time low, then you need not ponder that question ever again! It's mainly because diets put the dieter under the assumption that they can resume eating what they used to before their diet.

So now, you're at your goal weight, and you want to stay that way. It's a fact that the majority of Americans are overweight, so right now you just became a minority. I think it feels good to be among the successful group of dieters who have achieved their weight loss goals, and when you practice the proper weight maintenance strategy, you'll be a member of the elite dieters.

TOP TEN WAYS TO MAINTAIN YOUR WEIGHT LOSS

1. DETERMINE HOW MANY NET CALORIES YOU CAN CONSUME WHILE STILL MAINTAINING YOUR WEIGHT.

Here's a very simple way. If you have a fairly inactive lifestyle, and you're a middle-aged adult, take your current weight and multiply it by 12. That will tell you the approximate number of net calories you can eat each day and still maintain your current weight. There are bonuses if you exercise, because then you can multiply your body weight by 12 to 21, depending on your level of physical activity and your age. For example, if you exercise vigorously on a daily basis, then multiply your weight by 15, and that's how many net calories you can have each day.

Listed below are examples that will help you gauge your level of physical activity. Each unit represents 20 years of age beginning with the highest number for the lowest age increment.

Level of Exercise (Physical Activity)	Multiply your body weight by
Sedentary lifestyle with occasional exercise	18-12
1-3 times per week, light to moderate exercise	19-13
3-5 times per week, moderate to vigorous exercise	20-14
Daily exercise, moderate to vigorous	21-15

Let's see a real-life example of how much difference exercise can make for a 130-pound person:

Body Weight of Dieter	Daily Consumption
130 x 12	1,560 net calories
130 x 13	1,690 net calories
130 x 14	1,820 net calories
130 x 15	1,950 net calories

It's interesting to note the increase in net calories this dieter can eat if they simply exercise on a daily basis. This particular person could eat 390 more net calories per day by increasing their level of physical activity. The question you have to ask yourself is where your lifestyle fits into the maintenance equation. The good news is, now that you've learned to count your net calories, you'll be able to eat more because you're not counting any of the unabsorbed calories.

2.   DON'T LET THE WEIGHT CREEP BACK UP ON YOU.

Many dieters forget about the all-important weigh-in once they have achieved their weight loss goal. They tend to put less emphasis on their weight than when they weighed themselves on a regular basis to see how many pounds they lost that particular week. If you don't monitor your weight, how will you know if you're maintaining your weight loss? It's not a good idea to determine your weight by the way your clothes fit, because some people can wear the same clothes even after they've gained 10–15 pounds! It's a wise idea to weigh yourself at least once a week in order to monitor your progress. If you observe a weight gain, then it's time to reduce your net caloric intake in order to get back to your desired body weight. I weigh myself every day for several reasons. The first and foremost is that it shows me my daily weight fluctuation as a result of what I ate the previous day. In any case, you can't let one single weigh-in determine your diet destiny. If you become accustomed to your own individual weight fluctuations, then you'll be able to adjust your net caloric intake based on your average daily weight, not just a one-time final weigh-in.

The whole point here is to take control of your body weight and not let it control you. The sooner you discover that you're regaining weight, the quicker you can stop the process. Don't wait a month to step on the scale only to find that you've gained 10 pounds! The purpose of dieting is to lose weight and incorporate what you've learned into a daily routine so that you achieve permanent weight loss. It's vital to keep on top of the whole situation, and the best way to accomplish this is by monitoring your weight on a consistent basis.

Let me explain why you shouldn't let your weight fluctuate on a regular basis. It's a biological fact that when you quickly gain weight after dieting, the weight you put on is primarily comprised of fat (and some negligible water if you've been eating salty, processed foods). It's common for dieters who go on and off fad diets to lose and gain 20 pounds several times a year. Then they begin to wonder why they don't look the same as they used to, before their diet. Each time they gain their weight back, they look like they weigh even more than they used to. Their clothes fit tighter, and flab starts showing up in places that didn't seem to have that much body fat, like the triceps and back. The simple reason for this is that every time you gain weight back, it puts more pounds of fat on your figure. It's not advantageous to your appearance—or health—to quickly lose weight and then gain it back.

3. DETERMINE THAT THIS IS A GOAL YOU REALLY WANT TO KEEP!

Everyone starts a diet program for his or her own individual motives. It's common for dieters to lose weight for a special occasion such as a wedding, holiday event, or vacation. Another typical reason for dieting is to secure a date or spouse. Then there are the divorced dieters who are in search of true love once again. Whatever your inspiration was for dieting, the important thing is that it got you started, and now you've lost the weight. At this juncture, you need to ask yourself if the original prompt is still there, and if it isn't, then it's time to establish your own personal reasons why you need to maintain your weight loss.

It's time to get out a pen and paper and put your thoughts into words, which then become actions. It's time to make a commitment to yourself in writing. Now jot down at least five reasons or more why you want to stay at your desired weight.

The purpose of this lesson is to provide yourself with valid, concrete reasons for weight control and then refer to them when you feel like resorting back to your old eating habits. It's essential that you establish important motives, so you can incorporate them into your slim eating habits on a daily basis. If for some reason you're not ready to put them into written words, then ponder each one carefully and memorize them, so they can be recalled in times of dietary weakness.

4. DON'T KEEP YOUR DANGER FOODS IN THE HOUSE.

What I mean by danger foods are the types of food you used to eat that contributed to your weight gain in the first place. For instance, if you used to eat potato chips, cookies, and ice cream before you started dieting, then don't keep these things around, because they'll only tempt you to return to your old eating habits. If high-calorie food is readily available, there's a tendency to start munching on it and justifying the action by telling yourself that you're only going to eat a little bit. It doesn't matter how many excuses you drum up to eat these foods, because the calories add up much too quickly, and you'll end up gaining weight. If you start eating processed foods that contain artificial flavors, it will result in cravings that are much too difficult to control. Don't set yourself up for dietary disasters. If you absolutely must have "forbidden" food in the house, then the old adage "out of sight, out of mind" applies in this case. You should put the food where you don't see it or smell it so you're not lured into eating it.

5. I WANT TO STAY THIN IN A FAT SOCIAL GROUP.

It's time to take a good look around you and do a diet inventory. Recognize and count the number of people you associate with who are overweight. This includes co-workers, family, and friends. The primary reason for this inventory is to establish your diet friends and your diet foes (as was discussed in the Diet Buddies section).

You need to be ready for the typical remarks that will attempt to convince you to eat high-calorie food. The most common statements that are used to coerce you into a binge are listed below. For each one, a rebuttal is provided so you can assert yourself. Just personalize it to suit your situation.

Remark: You look great! One little dessert isn't going to make a difference.

Rebuttal: Thank you for the compliment, but I want to stay this way. The best way for me to do that is to abstain from eating my danger foods. I don't want one bite to lead to another, ending up with me gaining weight back, so I'll have something else instead.

Remark: You're thin. Why should you have to be concerned about what you eat?

Rebuttal: I appreciate your flattery, but the reason I'm thin is because I pay attention to the net calories I eat. If I ate whatever I wanted to, I would gain weight. I enjoy being thin more than I enjoy eating high-calorie food.

Remark: You've been dieting long enough. Why not live a little and eat something "good"? Go ahead and enjoy yourself. It's not every day you go to a party and have great appetizers and homemade cake.

Rebuttal: I've dieted long enough to know that I don't crave the high-calorie foods I used to eat when I was overweight. As a matter of fact, I will have some low-calorie appetizers because I saved up enough of my calories to eat some fruit with cheese and crackers. My tastes have changed, so what I think is good now is different from what I used to.

The moral of this diet lesson is that you need to be mentally prepared to deal with your peers and how they react to your successful weight loss. There are people who will try to convince you to break your diet. It happens on a daily basis. If you make up your mind in advance that you won't let other people determine what you eat, then you're ahead of the social games people play. It's time to show your friends and family that you've changed and that this isn't just a phase you're going through. If they've seen you lose and gain weight many times before, then they assume you'll repeat your past dieting performances. It's particularly rewarding to accomplish a goal when your peers think it's not achievable. If you stand in the presence of temptation and rise above it, then you will be stronger mentally, and saying no will become an automatic response instead of a learned behavior.

6. IT'S TIME TO DONATE YOUR LARGER-SIZED CLOTHES TO THE NEEDY OR A NON-PROFIT ORGANIZATION LIKE THE SALVATION ARMY, GOODWILL STORE, OR YOUR LOCAL CHURCH.

The main reason is so it won't be so convenient to gain weight and walk over to your closet and put on your larger clothes. One of my diet clients divulged to me that she has clothes that span ten sizes in her closet! She went on to explain that the reason is supposedly financial. If she gains weight, then she doesn't have to go out and buy a new wardrobe. I replied that keeping these clothes is like holding onto a piece of the past, and it makes a statement that's basically defeatist in nature. If you really want to stay normal weight, then why do you need your old clothes hanging about, unless you subconsciously plan to gain weight? It's similar to having an old pack of cigarettes in your house after you quit smoking. It's not a good idea to keep larger clothes in your closet that just sit there, waiting for you to gain weight. It's time to be firm in your decision to maintain your weight loss and throw away your dietary crutches—and walk away thin!

7. DON'T LET A DAY OF OVEREATING SABOTAGE YOUR WEIGHT MAINTENANCE.

This situation can be reversed simply by reducing your net caloric intake the next day. Your weight isn't determined by one day's eating but by your average consumption over time. For instance, suppose you normally consume 1,500 calories to maintain your weight, but one day you eat 2,000 calories. Now you've eaten 500 calories over your limit, but if you just subtract 250 calories for the next two days, you'll automatically lose that extra weight. So you should weigh yourself the morning after you overeat to see how much weight you've gained. This will help you determine how many days you should reduce your calories in order to get back to your desired weight.

If you avoid the scale because you've been overeating, you're only prolonging the inevitable. Ultimately you'll face the fact that you must reduce your net caloric intake in order to control your weight. It's important to take advantage of this system, because you don't want to keep losing and gaining weight. Your goal is to maintain your weight.

8. DON'T EAT FOODS WITHOUT KNOWING HOW MANY CALORIES THEY CONTAIN.

If a food item doesn't list the calories, it's because they're high. The food maker knows that divulging the truth about their calories will reduce their sales. The three biggest culprits of caloric secrecy are restaurants, bakeries, and farmers' markets. I'll give you a perfect example of how caloric ignorance causes weight gain. One of my clients was purchasing homemade cookies at her local farmers' market, and she estimated the calories to be about 150 calories each. I decided to investigate the situation because when she started eating them, she began to gain weight. I called the owner of the company, and he gave me the exact recipe with the contingency of confidentiality. I was happy to oblige, because I knew the information would validate my suspicion that these cookies were extremely high in calories. I proceeded to calculate the real calories of this mystery cookie and revealed the truth to my diet client. The cookie she counted as 150 calories was really 850 calories. If she ate only three of these cookies per week, it could result in a weight gain of 38 pounds by the end of the year!

It's always comforting to imagine that the calories are low, so you can justify eating the food, but the scale doesn't operate on guessed calories. It registers your weight based on your net calories. The best way to control your weight is to eat only the foods that list their calorie count on their labels.

9. YOU SHOULD GET AT LEAST 5 POUNDS BELOW YOUR GOAL WEIGHT.

There are two primary reasons for this, and the first of them is that it gives you some leeway in case you gain weight while you're on the maintenance stage of your diet program. This is similar to keeping extra money in your bank account just in case you spend more money than you anticipated. It's comforting to know that you have gone above and beyond your weight loss goal. This puts you into a positive frame of mind and prevents weight gain because you realize what you've accomplished. Now you're more determined and you have the confidence to maintain your weight.

The second rationale for getting below your goal weight is that most dieters realize that this magical number they've been striving for doesn't really leave them looking the way they wanted. You may be 40 years old, and your diet has brought you back to what you weighed at 30, but you could still look different in the mirror if your percentage of body fat is higher than it used to be. The best way to lower your body fat is by increasing your level of physical activity. One of the main benefits of reducing your body fat is that you'll look leaner (and thus thinner) than other people who weigh the same as you.

10. INCREASE YOUR LEVEL OF PHYSICAL ACTIVITY.

There are plenty of books written on the multitude of benefits you derive from daily exercise, so it's clearly advantageous to incorporate physical activity into your life every day. There are two significant reasons why regular exercise is essential to maintaining your weight loss. The first and foremost of these is the mere fact that you'll be able to consume more net calories and still control your weight. If you have a sedentary lifestyle, you'll have to consume fewer calories in order to stay at your goal weight. Since most dieters enjoy eating, the perfect way to give yourself caloric latitude is to burn additional calories by exercising.

It's important that you recognize that physical activity doesn't give you the right to eat everything and anything, because this attitude only sets you up for weight gain! You need to monitor your caloric intake in reference to your level of physical activity. Then you must weigh yourself to determine the impact of your exercise versus caloric consumption. The more you monitor yourself, the easier it is to maintain your weight.

The second basis for incorporating a daily exercise routine into your life is because it reminds your brain that physical exertion requires time and effort. Why would you want to work out for an hour and then eat all the calories you burned off by consuming one small sliver of pie? It's simply not worth it! When you exercise on a regular basis, it keeps you in a dieting frame of mind. You'll start noticing changes in your body, like a flatter stomach and firmer thighs, which inspire you to exercise more. This is the perfect time in your life to fine-tune your body and give yourself the look you've always wanted to achieve but lacked the confidence to make happen!

IN CLOSING

I've been contemplating this ending for quite some time. As Shakespeare once said, "Parting is such sweet sorrow." Then it came to me as I lay awake thinking. The reason that I started this program in the first place is what brought me to where I am today. I have a picture in my office of my husband and me. It sits on top of the bookshelf next to my hard-earned trophies. It's there to remind me of why I do what I do. It was taken at my diet client's wedding. Their photographer took it, and my diet client Maretta gave it to me as a token of her appreciation. I look at the smile on my face, knowing that there isn't enough money on earth to buy that kind of happiness. It wasn't my first diet client's wedding, and I'm positive there will be many more (p.s. I'll be happy to come if you invite me to your wedding).

Later that day I was racewalking in my neighborhood. I went past the house of Maretta's mom, Chris, and thought of how sweet it was that she helped me to type part of my manuscript so that I could rush it off to the publisher. She was on my diet at that time and offered to help me, without accepting anything but a thank you in return. My diet became part of their family's life. Maretta's mom and sister were both on my program. As I began the second half of my racewalk, a car pulled up to me. It was Maretta. She was smiling and waving and wanted to know when the book was coming out. As chance would have it, she moved into my neighborhood. She now has two darling children and a wonderful husband. She lost weight on my program, then married the man of her dreams.

As I came to the end of my racewalk, I thought, *It doesn't get any better than this!* I looked up at the beautiful blue sky as the cool breeze blew gently at the nape of my neck, providing relief from the heat of the summer sun. A song came to my mind that was perfect for the occasion. I've changed a word because it describes exactly how weight feels. "I can see clearly now, the weight is gone. It's gonna be a bright, bright, bright sunshiny day. Look straight ahead, nothing but blue skies." That's what lies ahead when you let your thin self out.

APPENDIX

FRUIT

25 Net Calories	Amount
Apricots	2
Blackberries	½ C.
Cantaloupe	¾ C.
Figs	1
Grapefruit	½
Guava	1
Kiwi	1
Peach	1
Persimmon	1
Plum	1
Quince	1 med.
Strawberries	½ C.
Tangerine	1
Watermelon	1 C.

50 Net Calories	Amount
Apple	1
Banana	1 med.
Blueberries	1 C.
Boysenberries	1 C.
Cherries	15
Elderberries	1 C.
Grapes	1 ¼ C.
Honeydew	1 C.
Mandarin orange	1
Mango	½ med.
Nectarine	1
Orange	1
Papaya	1 ¼ C.
Pear	1
Pineapple	1 C.
Pomegranate	1 med.
Raspberries	1 C.

VEGETABLES
25 NET CALORIE UNITS
R = RAW C = COOKED

	Amount
Alfalfa sprouts	12 C.
Artichoke hearts	½ C.

	Amount
Garden cress (r)	2 ¼ C.
Garden cress (c)	1 C.

Asparagus (r)	1 C.		Green beans	1 C.
Asparagus (c)	¾ C.		Kale (r)	5 C.
Avocado	1 sl.		Kohlrabi	¾ C.
Bamboo shoots (r)	1 C.		Leeks (r)	2 ¼ C.
Bamboo shoots (c)	1 C.		Leeks (c)	1 C.
Beets (r)	1 C.		Lettuce	5 C.
Beets (c)	¾ C.		Mung bean sprouts	3 C.
Broccoli (r)	1 ¼ C.		Mushrooms (all types) (r)	2 C.
Broccoli (c)	1 C.		Mushrooms (all types) (c)	1 C.
Brussels sprouts	½ C.		Mustard greens	3 C.
Cabbage (Chinese) (r)	5 C.		Okra	1 C.
Cabbage (Chinese) (c)	4 C.		Onions (r)	¾ C.
Cabbage (Green) (r)	5 C.		Onions (c)	½ C.
Cabbage (Green) (c)	4C.		Peppers, hot	1 ¼ C.
Cabbage (Red) (r)	5 C.		Peppers, sweet (green, red) (r)	1 ¾ C.
Cabbage (Red) (c)	4C.		Peppers, sweet (green, red) (c)	1 1/3 C.
Cabbage (Savoy) (r)	5 C.		Pumpkin (c)	1 C.
Cabbage (Savoy) (c)	4 C.		Squash (summer) (c)	1 C.
Carrots (r)	¾ C.		Squash (zucchini) (r)	2 ½ C.
Carrots (c)	½ C.		Squash (zucchini) (c)	1 1/3 C.
Cauliflower (r)	1 ½ C.		Swamp Cabbage (r)	3 ¼ C.
Cauliflower (c)	1 C.		Swamp Cabbage (c)	1 ¾ C.
Celeriac	½ C.		Tomato (r)	1 ¼ C.
Celery	10 stalks		Tomato (c)	½ C.
Chard (Swiss)	2 C.		Turnip (c)	1 ¼ C.
Collards	4 C.		Turnip Greens (r)	4 C.
Cucumber	2 ½ C.		Turnip Greens (c)	1 C.
Dandelion greens (r)	5 C.		Water Chestnuts raw or boiled	½ C.
Dandelion greens (c)	2 C.		Water cress	9 C.
Eggplant (c)	1 ½ C.		Wax Beans (c)	1 C.
Endive	5 C.			

100 NET CALORIE UNITS OF COMMON FOODS
R = RAW C = COOKED

	Amount		Amount
Adzuki Beans (c)	½ C.	Parsnips (c)	1 ¼ C.
Baked Beans (vegetarian) (c)	¾ C.	Peas (r)	1 ½ C.
Beans, Refried (Fat Free) (c)	¾ C.	Peas (c)	1 C.
Black Beans (c)	¾ C.	Peas (split) (c)	1 C.
Black Turtle Beans (c)	¾ C.	Pink Beans (c)	¾ C.
Broad bean (c)	1 C.	Pinto Beans (c)	¾ C.
Butterbean (c)	¾ C.	Potato (c)	1 C.
Cannellini Beans (c)	1 C.	Red Beans (c)	¾ C.
Chick Peas (Garbanzo) (c)	¾ C.	Rice, Brown (c)	¾ C.
Corn (c)	1 ½ C.	Soybeans, Green (c)	¾ C.
Cow Peas (black-eyed peas) (c)	¾ C.	Soybeans (c)	¾ C.
Cranberry Beans (c)	1 C.	Squash, acorn (c)	1 ¼ C.
Fava Beans (c)	¾ C.	Squash, butternut (c)	1 ¼ C.
Great Northern Beans (c)	¾ C.	Squash, Hubbard (c)	2 C.
Kidney Beans (c)	¾ C.	Squash, Spaghetti (c)	3 ½ C.
Lentils (c)	1 C.	Succotash (c)	1 C.
Lima Beans (c)	¾ C.	Sweet Potato (c)	¾ C.
Lupin Beans (c)	¾ C.	Taro (c)	¾ C.
Mung Beans (c)	¾ C.	White Beans (c)	¾ C.
Navy Beans (c)	¾ C.	Yam (c)	1 ½ C.

NUTS, SEEDS, AND NUT BUTTERS

Acorn, raw	1 oz.	60	Peanut butter, smooth raw	1 oz.	64
Almond butter, raw	1 Tbsp.	70	Peanut butter, roasted w/o oil	1 Tbsp.	72
Almond butter, roasted w/o oil	1 Tbsp.	80	Peanut butter roasted w/oil	1 Tbsp.	86
Almond butter, roasted w / oil	1 Tbsp.	90	Peanut butter, raw crunchy	1 Tbsp.	72

Almonds, raw	1 oz.	102	Peanut butter, crunchy, roasted	1 Tbsp.	76
Almonds, dry roasted	1 oz.	136	Peanut butter, roasted w/oil	1 Tbsp.	90
Almonds, roasted in oil	1 oz.	162	Peanuts, boiled	1 oz.	81
Brazil nuts, raw	1 oz.	108	Peanuts, raw	1 oz.	100
Brazil nuts, roasted w/o oil	1 oz.	144	Peanuts, roasted w/o oil	1 oz.	136
Brazil nuts, roasted in oil	1 oz.	162	Peanuts, roasted w/oil	1 oz.	153
Cashews, raw	1 oz.	100	Pecan butter, raw	1 Tbsp.	80
Cashews, roasted w/o oil	1 oz.	134	Pecan butter, roasted w/o oil	1 Tbsp.	88
Cashews, roasted in oil	1 oz.	153	Pecan butter roasted w/oil	1 Tbsp.	99
Cashew butter, raw	1 Tbsp.	56	Pecans, raw	1 oz.	114
Cashew butter, roasted w/o oil	1 Tbsp.	64	Pecans, roasted w/o oil	1 oz.	152
Cashew butter roasted w/oil	1 Tbsp.	72	Pecans roasted in oil	1 oz.	180
Chinese chestnuts, raw	1 oz.	38	Pine nuts, dried	1 oz.	88
Chinese chestnuts, boiled	1 oz.	30	Pistachio nuts, raw	1 oz.	96
Chinese chestnuts, dried	1 oz.	82	Pistachio nuts roasted w/o oil	1 oz.	137
Chinese chestnut, dry roasted	1 oz.	61	Pistachio nuts roasted in oil	1 oz.	153
European chestnuts, raw	1 oz.	36	Pumpkin seeds, raw	1 oz.	96
European, chestnuts, boiled	1 oz.	30	Pumpkin seeds, roasted w/o oil	1 oz.	136
European chestnuts, dried	1 oz.	84	Pumpkin seeds roasted in oil	1 oz.	153
European chestnuts, roasted	1 oz.	63	Sesame seeds, raw	1 oz.	96
Japanese chestnuts, raw	1 oz.	27	Sesame seeds roasted w/o oil	1 oz.	128
Japanese chestnuts, boiled	1 oz.	12	Sesame seeds roasted in oil	1 oz.	144
Japanese chestnuts, dried	1 oz.	81	Sesame butter, raw	1 Tbsp.	67

Japanese chestnuts, roasted	1 oz.	45	Sesame butter roasted w/o oil	1 Tbsp.	72
Coconut, raw	1 oz.	60	Sesame butter roasted w/ oil	1 oz.	81
Coconut, shredded w/o sugar	2 Tbsp.	64	Soy nuts, raw	1 oz.	70
Filberts. Raw	1 oz.	105	Soy nuts, roasted w/o oil	1 oz.	103
Filberts, roasted w/o oil	1 oz.	143	Soy nuts, roasted in oil	1 oz.	113
Filberts, roasted in oil	1 oz.	168	Soy nut butter, roasted w/o oil	1 Tbsp.	64
Ginkgo nuts, raw	1 oz.	32	Sunflower seeds, raw	1 oz.	89
Ginkgo nuts, dried w/o oil	1 oz.	79	Sunflower seeds roasted w/o oil	1 oz.	134
Hickory nuts, dried w/o oil	1 oz.	150	Sunflower seeds roasted in oil	1 oz.	151
Macadamia nuts, dried	1 oz.	159	Walnut butter, raw	1 Tbsp.	77
Macadamia nuts, w/o oil	1 oz.	154	Walnut butter roasted w/o oil	1 Tbsp.	84
Macadamia nuts, w/oil	1 oz.	184	Walnut butter roasted w/oil	1 Tbsp.	94
Mixed nuts, raw	1 oz.	102	Walnuts, raw	1 oz.	114
Mixed nuts roasted w/oil	1 oz.	135	Walnuts, roasted w/o oil	1 oz.	156
Mixed nuts roasted in oil	1 oz.	160	Walnuts, roasted in oil	1 oz.	176

The Who Chart			
Diet Saboteur	Current Weight Condition Overweight = OW Normal weight = NW Gaining Weight = GW	Are They Dieting? Yes = Y No =N	What was your response when they asked you to eat?
1			
2			
3			
4			
5			
6			

7			
8			
9			
10			

The What Chart (Snack Foods)			
Crunchy, Salty group		**Smooth, Sweet group**	
High Calorie Type	Lower Calorie option	High Calorie Type	Lower Calorie option
1		1	
2		2	
3		3	
4		4	
5		5	
6		6	
7		7	
8		8	
9		9	
10		10	

The Where Chart
Top 10 places I tend to overeat (restaurant, Grandma's house, buffet, parties, etc)
1
2
3
4
5
6
7
8
9
10

DIETARY OBSERVATION CHART

KEY:

1 = I ate because it was breakfast

2 = I ate because it was lunchtime

3 = I ate because it was dinnertime

4 = I ate because it was snack time

5 = I ate because I saw someone eating

6 = I ate because I was bored

7 = I ate because I was offered food

8 = I ate because my children were

9 = I ate because I was in a bad mood

10 = I ate to relieve stress

11 = I ate because I saw food on TV

12 = I had the urge to eat but did not

The When Chart							
Time	Monday	Tuesday	Wednesday	Thursday	Friday	Saturday	Sunday
	Key 0-12	Key 0-12	Key 0-12	Key 0-12	Key 0-12	Key 0-12	Key 0-12
7:00-8:00 a.m.							
8:00-9:00							
9:00-10:00							
10:00-11:00							
11:00-12:00 p.m.							
12:00-1:00							
1:00-2:00							
2:00-3:00							

3:00-4:00							
4:00-5:00							
5:00-6:00							
6:00-7:00							
7:00-8:00							
8:00-9:00							
9:00-10:00							
10:00-11:00							
11:00p.m. -7:00 a.m.							

The Why Chart	
Food that I overeat	Why I consume this type of food

e|LIVE

listen|imagine|view|experience

AUDIO BOOK DOWNLOAD INCLUDED WITH THIS BOOK!

In your hands you hold a complete digital entertainment package. Besides purchasing the paper version of this book, this book includes a free download of the audio version of this book. Simply use the code listed below when visiting our website. Once downloaded to your computer, you can listen to the book through your computer's speakers, burn it to an audio CD or save the file to your portable music device (such as Apple's popular iPod) and listen on the go!

How to get your free audio book digital download:

1. Visit www.tatepublishing.com and click on the e|LIVE logo on the home page.
2. Enter the following coupon code:
   1e83-a4fa-184f-ade0-146f-8547-9a1a-13ec
3. Download the audio book from your e|LIVE digital locker and begin enjoying your new digital entertainment package today!